A POCKET MANUAL OF DIFFERENTIAL DIAGNOSIS

W9-AAZ-092

Haleh

A POCKET MANUAL OF DIFFERENTIAL DIAGNOSIS

Third Edition

Stephen N. Adler, M.D.
Clinical Instructor in Medicine, University of Oklahoma
College of Medicine; Medical Director, Respiratory
Therapy, Mercy Health Center and Deaconess Hospital,
Oklahoma City

Mildred Lam, M.D.
Associate Professor of Medicine, Case Western Reserve
University School of Medicine; Staff Physician, Division of
Nephrology, MetroHealth Medical Center, Cleveland

Dianne B. Gasbarra, M.D.
Clinical Instructor in Medicine, University of Oklahoma
College of Medicine; Chairman, Department of Pulmonary
Medicine, Mercy Health Center, Oklahoma City

Alfred F. Connors, Jr., M.D.
Associate Professor of Medicine, Case Western Reserve
University School of Medicine; Director, Medical Intensive
Care Unit, MetroHealth Medical Center, Cleveland

Little, Brown and Company
Boston   New York   Toronto   London

To Our Parents

Copyright © 1994 by Stephen N. Adler, Mildred Lam, Dianne B. Gasbarra, and Alfred F. Connors, Jr.

Third Edition

Previous editions copyright © 1982 by Little, Brown and Company (Inc.); 1988 by Stephen N. Adler, Mildred Lam, Dianne B. Gasbarra, and Alfred F. Connors, Jr.

Library of Congress Cataloging-in-Publication Data

A pocket manual of differential diagnosis / Stephen N. Adler . . . [et al.].—3rd ed.
        p.   cm.
    Includes bibliographical references and index.
    ISBN 0-316-01109-6
    1. Diagnosis, Differential—Handbooks, manuals, etc.
I. Adler, Stephen N.
    [DNLM: 1. Diagnosis, Differential—handbooks.
WB 39 P739 1994]
RC71.5.A34   1994
616.07'5—dc20
DNLM/DLC
for Library of Congress   93-33819
                                                                CIP

Printed in the United States of America

KP

Editorial: Laurie Anello
Production Editor/Copyeditor: Marie A. Salter
Indexer: Nancy Newman
Production Supervisor: Cate Rickard
Cover Designer: Rogalski Associates

CONTENTS

3. Drugs 61
Stephen N. Adler

4. Endocrine/Metabolic System 103
Thomas A. Murphy

5. Eye 139
Mildred Lam

6. Gastrointestinal and Hepatic Systems 153
Wendell K. Clarkston and Bruce R, Bacon

CONTRIBUTING AUTHORS

David J. Adelstein, M.D.
Staff Physician, Department of Hematology and Oncology, Cleveland Clinic Foundation, Cleveland

Stephen N. Adler, M.D.
Clinical Instructor in Medicine, University of Oklahoma College of Medicine; Medical Director, Respiratory Therapy, Mercy Health Center and Deaconess Hospital, Oklahoma City

Bruce R. Bacon, M.D.
Professor of Internal Medicine, St. Louis University School of Medicine; Director, Division of Gastroenterology and Hepatology, St. Louis University Health Sciences Center, St. Louis

Wendell K. Clarkston, M.D.
Assistant Professor of Internal Medicine, St. Louis University School of Medicine; Staff Physician, Division of Gastroenterology and Hepatology, St. Louis University Health Sciences Center, St. Louis

Alfred F. Connors, Jr., M.D.
Associate Professor of Medicine, Case Western Reserve University School of Medicine; Director, Medical Intensive Care Unit, MetroHealth Medical Center, Cleveland

Dianne B. Gasbarra, M.D.
Clinical Instructor in Medicine, University of Oklahoma College of Medicine; Chairman, Department of Pulmonary Medicine, Mercy Health Center, Oklahoma City

Mildred Lam, M.D.
Associate Professor of Medicine, Case Western Reserve University School of Medicine; Staff Physician, Division of Nephrology, MetroHealth Medical Center, Cleveland

Thomas A. Murphy, M.D.
Assistant Professor of Medicine, Case Western Reserve University School of Medicine; Director, Division of Endocrinology, MetroHealth Medical Center, Cleveland

PREFACE

In the practice of clinical medicine, one encounters a variety of symptoms, signs, and laboratory tests. Each clinical finding and test result is associated with a differential diagnosis; that is, a list of conditions or disease entities that can produce the given finding or result. Differential diagnoses for various clinical findings are readily available in medical texts and other sources, but the information is often scattered in a number of different references. Our book contains information gathered from many such sources, but it is compiled in a compact form. It therefore serves as a convenient guide in the workup of clinical problems and is a valuable teaching tool as well. Intended for medical students, physician's assistants, house officers, and practicing and teaching clinicians, this book helps make the process of medical diagnosis more efficient and comprehensive. It does not, however, serve as a substitute for the thoughtful, skillful integration of data obtained by careful history-taking, physical examination, and judicious use of laboratory tests.

A Pocket Manual of Differential Diagnosis, Third Edition, has been thoroughly reviewed and updated. The recent explosion of new pharmaceutical agents has mandated major changes in the text particularly with respect to therapeutics, including drug toxicities. Because of the widespread impact of AIDS on modern medicine, every effort has been made to include the most current information available on the manifestations and complications of this disease.

The text is again divided into 13 chapters, ten of which are organized by organ system; the remaining three discuss acid-base and electrolyte disorders, drugs, and infectious disease. Each chapter contains multiple entries, representing symptoms, clinical signs, laboratory tests, radiologic findings, and disease processes; 193 separate entries compose the text. The differential diagnosis for each entry is listed, with more common disease entities generally being listed first; extremely rare entities or those of questionable documentation are often omitted. Where possible, disease entities are organized by pathophysiologic mechanism. At the end of each entry, references, usually general or subspecialty texts, are listed. Entries are cross-referenced, and the book is indexed. A bibliography of general and subspecialty texts is also included at the end of the book.

We acknowledge the expert secretarial assistance of Fran Apitauer, Pat Garnett, Connie Jones, Anne LaGania, Joan Skiba, Shari Venable, and Teresa Greenhill. We are also grateful to our editors, Laurie Anello and Marie Salter, of Little, Brown, who helped prepare this edition. Finally, we give special acknowledgment to the housestaff and medical students of the Case Western Reserve medical community, and of the University of Oklahoma Health Sciences Center, whose support and encouragement have made preparation of this third edition worthwhile.

S.N.A.
M.L.
D.B.G.
A.F.C.

A POCKET
MANUAL OF
DIFFERENTIAL
DIAGNOSIS

Notice

The indications and dosages of all drugs in this book have been recommended in the medical literature and conform to the practices of the general medical community. The medications described do not necessarily have specific approval by the Food and Drug Administration for use in the diseases and dosages for which they are recommended. The package insert for each drug should be consulted for use and dosage as approved by the FDA. Because standards for usage change, it is advisable to keep abreast of revised recommendations, particularly those concerning new drugs.

1 ACID-BASE AND ELECTROLYTE DISORDERS

1-A. Acid-Base Nomogram

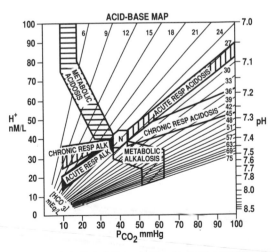

Source: Goldberg M, et al: Computer-Based Instruction and Diagnosis of Acid-Base Disorders. *JAMA* 223:270, 1973. Copyright © 1973 by the American Medical Association.

1-B. Metabolic Acidosis

Increased Anion Gap
Renal failure, acute or chronic
Ketoacidosis
  Diabetic
  Alcoholic
  Starvation
Lactic acidosis (see 1-E)
Toxins
  Aspirin
  Methanol
  Ethylene glycol
  Paraldehyde
  Toluene
Nonketotic hyperosmolar coma
Inborn errors of metabolism (e.g., maple syrup urine disease, methylmalonic aciduria)

Normal Anion Gap
Gastrointestinal loss
  Diarrhea
  Ileal loop, ureterosigmoidostomy
  Small-bowel or pancreatic fistula or drainage
  Anion-exchange resins (e.g., cholestyramine)
  Calcium or magnesium chloride ingestion
Renal loss
  Renal tubular acidosis (see 7-F)
  Hypoaldosteronism
  Carbonic anhydrase inhibitors
Recovery phase of ketoacidosis
Rapid expansion of extracellular fluid volume with bicarbonate-free fluid (e.g., dilutional acidosis)
Hyperalimentation with excess of cationic amino acids
Acidifying agents (e.g., ammonium chloride, arginine hydrochloride, lysine hydrochloride)
Sulfur ingestion

References
1. Shapiro JI, Kaehny WD: Pathogenesis and Management of Metabolic Acidosis and Alkalosis. In general reference 16, p 161.
2. Narins RG, Krishna GG, Bressler L: The Metabolic Acidoses. In general reference 6, p 597.

1-C. Respiratory Acidosis

Neuromuscular Causes

Ingestion or overdose (e.g., tranquilizers, sedatives, anes-
thetics, anticholinesterases)
Cerebral, brainstem, or high spinal-cord injury or infarct
Primary neuromuscular disease
  Guillain-Barré syndrome
  Myasthenia gravis
  Amyotrophic lateral sclerosis
  Poliomyelitis
  Botulism
  Tetanus
Myopathy involving respiratory muscles, especially:
  Muscular dystrophy
  Hypokalemic myopathy
  Familial periodic paralysis
Primary hypoventilation
Sleep apnea syndrome
Diaphragmatic paralysis

Airway Obstruction

Upper airway
  Laryngeal edema or spasm
  Tracheal edema, stenosis
  Obstructive sleep apnea
Lower airway
  Mechanical
    Foreign body
    Aspirated fluid (e.g., vomitus)
    Neoplasm
  Bronchospasm
    Acute
    Chronic (e.g., chronic obstructive pulmonary disease)

Cardiopulmonary-Thoracic Causes

Cardiac arrest
Severe pneumonia
Severe pulmonary edema
Respiratory distress syndrome (infant or adult)
Restrictive lung disease (e.g., interstitial fibrosis)
Massive pulmonary embolism
Pneumothorax, hemothorax
Chest trauma
Kyphoscoliosis

Smoke inhalation
Improper mechanical ventilation

References
1. Gennari FJ: Respiratory Acidosis and Alkalosis. In general reference 6, p 713.
2. Kaehny WD: Pathogenesis and Management of Respiratory and Mixed Acid-Base Disorders. In general reference 16, p 211.

1-D. Anion Gap

Increased
Without acidosis
    Administration of sodium salts of organic compounds
        (e.g., citrate, lactate, acetate)
    High-dose penicillin or carbenicillin
    Respiratory or metabolic alkalosis
    Dehydration
With acidosis
    Renal failure, acute or chronic
    Ketoacidosis
      Diabetic
      Starvation
      Alcoholic
    Nonketotic hyperosmolar coma
    Lactic acidosis (see 1-E)
    Toxins
      Aspirin
      Methanol
      Ethylene glycol
      Paraldehyde
      Toluene
    Inborn errors of metabolism

Decreased
Hypoalbuminemia
Hypernatremia, severe
Dilution of extracellular fluid
Multiple myeloma
Hyperviscosity
Bromide ingestion
Hypercalcemia, hypermagnesemia (severe)
Lithium toxicity

References
1. Emmett M, Narins RG: Clinical Use of the Anion Gap. *Medicine* 56:38, 1977.
2. Oh MS, Carroll HJ: Current Concepts: The Anion Gap. *N Engl J Med* 297:814, 1977.

1-E. Lactic Acidosis

Associated with Impaired Tissue Oxygenation (Type A)
Shock (e.g., hypovolemic, cardiogenic, septic)
Hypoxemia, respiratory failure
Anemia, severe

Occurring in Absence of Apparent Hypoxemia or Circulatory Insufficiency (Type B)
Diabetes, uncontrolled
Hepatic failure
Renal failure
Malignancy, especially leukemia or lymphoma
Drugs, toxins
  Cyanide
  Carbon monoxide
  Methanol
  Salicylates
  Iron
  Strychnine
  Ethanol
Seizures
Excessive muscular activity (e.g., excessive exercise)
Alkalosis, respiratory or metabolic
D-Lactic acidosis (secondary to intestinal bacterial overgrowth)
Congenital enzyme deficiency (e.g, glycogen storage disease)

References
1. Shapiro JI, Kaehny WD: Pathogenesis and Management of Metabolic Acidosis and Alkalosis. In general reference 16, p 161.
2. Narins RG, Krishhna GG, Bressler L, et al: The Metabolic Acidoses. In general reference 6, p 597.
3. Kreisberg RA: Lactate Homeostasis and Lactic Acidosis. *Ann Intern Med* 92:227, 1980.

1-F. Metabolic Alkalosis

Chloride-Responsive (Urine Cl⁻ < 10 mEq/L)
Vomiting, nasogastric suction
Gastric drainage or fistula
Diuretics
Posthypercapnic state
Villous adenoma of colon
Congenital chloride diarrhea
Cystic fibrosis

Chloride-Resistant (Urine Cl⁻ > 20 mEq/L)
Primary aldosteronism
Secondary aldosteronism
  Congestive heart failure
  Cirrhosis and ascites
  Malignant hypertension
  Adrenocorticotropic hormone (ACTH) or glucocorticoid
      excess (Cushing's disease, Cushing's syndrome, ec-
      topic ACTH production)
  Bartter's syndrome
  Renin-secreting tumor (e.g., hemangiopericytoma)
Licorice ingestion
Excessive use of chewing tobacco
Severe potassium depletion
Congenital adrenal hyperplasia
Liddle's syndrome

Miscellaneous
Administration of alkali or alkalinizing agents, especially in
    the presence of renal insufficiency:
  Alkalinizing agents (e.g., citrate, lactate)
  Antacids (milk-alkali syndrome)
  Massive transfusion of blood or plasma substitute
Nonparathyroid hypercalcemia (e.g., bone metastases,
    multiple myeloma)
Nonreabsorbable anionic antibiotics, large doses (e.g.,
    penicillin, carbenicillin)
Glucose ingestion after starvation

References
1. Shapiro JI, Kaehny WD: Pathogenesis and Management
   of Metabolic Acidosis and Alkalosis. In general reference
   16, p 161.
2. Sabatini S, Kurtzman NA: Metabolic Alkalosis. In general
   reference 6, p 691.

1-G. Respiratory Alkalosis

Central Causes
Voluntary hyperventilation
Anxiety, pain
Hypoxia
Fever
Salicylate toxicity
Head trauma
Brain tumor
Central nervous system infection
Cerebrovascular accident
Pregnancy
Recovery phase of metabolic acidosis

Cardiopulmonary Causes
Congestive heart failure
Pneumonia
Pulmonary embolism
Interstitial lung disease
Adult respiratory distress syndrome
High altitude

Other
Hepatic insufficiency
Sepsis (especially gram-negative)
Drugs
   Progesterone, medroxyprogesterone
   Xanthines (e.g., aminophylline)
   Catecholamines (massive amounts)
   Nicotine
Mechanical ventilation
Heat exposure (e.g., heat stroke)

References
1. Cohen JJ, Kassirer JP: Acid-Base Metabolism. In general reference 6, p 181.
2. Kaehny WD: Pathogenesis and Management of Respiratory and Mixed Acid-Base Disorders. In general reference 16, p 211.

1-H. Hypernatremia

Pure Water Loss
Inability to obtain or swallow water (e.g., coma, dementia, infancy)
Impaired thirst drive (e.g., hypothalamic lesion)
Increased insensible loss

Excessive Sodium Intake
Iatrogenic sodium administration
  Sodium bicarbonate (cardiac arrest, treatment of lactic acidosis)
  Hypertonic saline (therapeutic abortion)
Accidental or deliberate ingestion of large quantities of sodium (e.g., substitution of salt for sugar in infant formula)
Seawater ingestion or drowning
Mineralocorticoid or glucocorticoid excess
  Primary aldosteronism
  Cushing's syndrome
  Ectopic adrenocorticotropic hormone production

Loss of Water in Excess of Sodium (Without Concomitant Water Intake)
Gastrointestinal loss (e.g., vomiting, diarrhea, intestinal fistula)
Renal loss
  Central diabetes insipidus
    Head trauma
    Posthypophysectomy
    Tumor
    Granulomatous disease (e.g., sarcoidosis, tuberculosis, Wegener's granulomatosis, syphilis, histiocytosis)
    Central nervous system infection
    Vascular lesion (e.g., cerebrovascular accident, aneurysm, sickle cell disease, Sheehan's syndrome)
    Congenital
  Impaired renal concentrating ability
    Osmotic diuresis
      Diabetic ketoacidosis
      Chronic renal failure, especially interstitial disease (e.g., polycystic disease, medullary cystic disease)
      Partial urinary tract obstruction, postobstructive diuresis
      Diuretic phase of acute renal failure
      Mannitol

Tube feedings
Infant formula (especially cow's milk)
Excessive diuretic use
Hypokalemia
Hypercalcemia
Decreased protein intake
Prolonged, excessive water intake
Sickle cell disease or trait
Multiple myeloma
Amyloidosis
Sarcoidosis
Sjögren's syndrome
Nephrogenic diabetes insipidus, congenital

Drugs
Alcohol
Lithium
Demeclocycline
Phenytoin
Propoxyphene
Sulfonylurea hypoglycemic agents
Amphotericin B
Methoxyflurane
Colchicine
Vinblastine
Skin loss (e.g., burns, sweating)
Peritoneal dialysis

Essential Hypernatremia (Reset Osmostat)

References
1. Ross EJ, Christie SBM: Hypernatremia. *Medicine*
   48:441, 1969.
2. Berl T, Schrier RW: Disorders of Water Metabolism. In
   general reference 16, p 1.

1-I. Hyponatremia

Factitious Hyponatremia (Normal Serum Osmolality)
Hyperglycemia
Hyperlipidemia
Hyperproteinemia
Hypertonic infusion of poorly reabsorbed solute (e.g., mannitol)

States with Decreased Extracellular Fluid Volume (Loss of Hypotonic Fluid Coupled with Water Intake)

Gastrointestinal loss (e.g., vomiting, diarrhea)

Third-space loss (e.g., burns, sweating, hemorrhagic pancreatitis)

Renal loss

Diuretic use

    Renal salt-wasting (e.g., advanced chronic renal failure, interstitial disease, renal tubular acidosis)

    Osmotic diuresis

    Mineralocorticoid deficiency

States with Increased Extracellular Fluid Volume

Congestive heart failure

Cirrhosis and ascites

Nephrotic syndrome

Renal failure, acute or chronic

States with Normal or Slightly Increased Extracellular Fluid Volume

Syndrome of inappropriate antidiuretic hormone (SIADH)

    Central nervous system disease

        Tumor

        Trauma

        Infection (meningitis, encephalitis, abscess)

        Cerebrovascular accident (thrombosis or hemorrhage)

        Guillain-Barré syndrome

        Delirium tremens

        Multiple sclerosis

    Pulmonary disease

        Tumor

        Pneumonia

        Lung abscess

        Tuberculosis

    Carcinoma (especially lung, pancreas, duodenum)

    Pain, stress (e.g., postoperative state)

    Acute psychosis

Adrenal insufficiency $\downarrow Na$

    Hypothyroidism

    Positive-pressure ventilation

    Porphyria

Drugs

    Antidiuretic hormone and analogues

    Nicotine

    Sulfonylurea compounds (especially chlorpropamide)

    Morphine

Barbiturates
Isoproterenol
Nonsteroidal antiinflammatory drugs
Acetaminophen
Clofibrate
Carbamazepine
Phenothiazines (thioridazine, fluphenazine)
Amitriptyline
Colchicine
Vincristine
Cyclophosphamide
Psychogenic polydipsia with massive water intake (> 20–25 L/day)
Beer drinking (excessive) associated with malnutrition
Essential (reset osmostat)

References
1. Berl T, Schrier RW: Disorders of Water Metabolism. In general reference 16, p 1.
2. Rossi NF, Schrier RW: Hyponatremic States. In general reference 6, p 461.

1-J. Hyperkalemia

Pseudohyperkalemia
Tourniquet use
Hemolysis (in vitro)
Leukocytosis, thrombocytosis

Intracellular-to-Extracellular K^+ Shift
Acidosis
Heavy exercise
Beta-blocking agents
Insulin deficiency
Digitalis intoxication
Hyperkalemic periodic paralysis

K^+ Load (Especially in Presence of Renal Insufficiency)
K^+ supplements
K^+-rich foods
K^+-containing salt substitute
Intravenous K^+
K^+-containing drugs (e.g., potassium penicillin)

Transfusion of aged blood
Hemolysis
Gastrointestinal bleeding
Cell destruction post-chemotherapy (especially with leukemia, lymphoma, myeloma)
Rhabdomyolysis or crush injury
Extensive tissue necrosis or catabolic state

Decreased K⁺ Excretion

Renal failure (acute or chronic)
Drugs
  K^+-sparing diuretics (spironolactone, triamterene, amiloride)
  Beta-blocking agents
  Nonsteroidal antiinflammatory drugs
  Converting enzyme inhibitors (e.g., captopril)
Aldosterone deficiency (see 7-F, Renal Tubular Acidosis, Type IV)
Selective defect in renal K^+ excretion
  Pseudohypoaldosteronism
  Lupus erythematosus
  Sickle cell disease
  Obstructive uropathy
  Renal transplantation
  Congenital

References

1. DeFronzo RA: Hyperkalemic States. In general reference 6, p 547.
2. Gabow PA, Peterson LN: Disorders of Potassium Metabolism. In general reference 16, p 231.

1-K. Hypokalemia

Extracellular-to-intracellular K^+ shifts
  Alkalosis
  Increased plasma insulin (e.g., treatment phase of diabetic ketoacidosis)
  Beta-adrenergic agonists
  Hypokalemic periodic paralysis
creased intake
  oor dietary intake
  ophagia

Gastrointestinal loss
  Vomiting, nasogastric suction
  Diarrhea, laxative or enema abuse
  Malabsorption
  Ureterosigmoidostomy, ileal loop
  Enteric fistula
  Villous adenoma
Renal loss
  Diuretic therapy
  Primary aldosteronism
  Secondary aldosteronism
    Malignant hypertension
    Renal artery stenosis
    Congestive heart failure
    Cirrhosis and ascites
    Adrenocorticotropic hormone (ACTH) or glucocorticoid
      excess (Cushing's disease, Cushing's syndrome, ec-
      topic ACTH production)
    Bartter's syndrome
    Renin-secreting tumor (e.g., renal hemangiopericy-
      toma)
  Licorice ingestion
  Excessive use of chewing tobacco
  Renal tubular acidosis
  Diuresis during recovery from obstruction or acute renal
    failure
  Osmotic diuresis
  Drugs and toxins
    Carbenicillin, penicillin (large doses)
    Amphotericin B
    L-Dopa
    Lithium
    Thallium
  Hypomagnesemia
  Acute leukemia
  Congenital adrenal hyperplasia
Sweat loss
  Heavy exercise
  Heat stroke
States of rapid cellular synthesis
  Intravenous hyperalimentation
  Recovery from megaloblastic anemia

References
1. Raymond KH, Kunan RT: Hypokalemic States. In general
   reference 6, p 519.
2. Gabow PA, Peterson LN: Disorders of Potassium Metabolism. In general reference 16, p 231.

1-L. Hypercalcemia

Hemoconcentration (increased serum albumin)*
Hyperparathyroidism
  Primary
    Parathyroid adenoma
    Parathyroid hyperplasia
    Parathyroid carcinoma
    Multiple endocrine adenomatosis
  Secondary (e.g., chronic renal failure)
  Ectopic
Malignancy
  Bony metastases
  Humoral factors (e.g., parathyroid hormone–like sub-
    stances, osteoclast activating factor)
  Calcium-binding globulin (multiple myeloma)*
Thiazide diuretics
Immobilization (in association with rapid bone turnover
    states, e.g., adolescence or Paget's disease)
Milk-alkali syndrome
Vitamin D intoxication
Vitamin A intoxication
Granulomatous disease (especially sarcoidosis, tuberculo-
    sis)
Hypophosphatemia
Recovery from rhabdomyolysis-induced acute renal failure
Hyperthyroidism
Adrenal insufficiency
Acromegaly
Lithium administration
Familial hypocalciuric hypercalcemia
Idiopathic infantile hypercalcemia
Blue-diaper syndrome
Hypophosphatasia
Metaphyseal chondrodysplasia

References

1. Benabe JE, Martinez-Maldonado M: Disorders of Calcium Metabolism. In general reference 6, p 759.
2. Popovtzer MM, Knochel JP, Kumar R: Disorders of Calcium, Phosphorus, Vitamin D, and Parathyroid Hormone
   Activity. In general reference 16, p 287.

*Normal serum ionized calcium.

1-M. Hypocalcemia

Hypoalbuminemia*
Vitamin D deficiency states
  Sunlight deficiency
  Dietary deficiency
  Malabsorption (see 6-G)
    Postgastrectomy
    Sprue
    Pancreatic insufficiency
    Hepatobiliary disease with bile salt deficiency
    Laxative abuse
  Abnormal metabolism of vitamin D
    Renal failure (acute and chronic)
    Liver failure
    Vitamin D–dependent rickets
    Anticonvulsants, microsomal enzyme inducers
Hypoparathyroidism
  Congenital
  Idiopathic (infantile and adolescent-onset types)
  Acquired
    Surgical
    Iron overload (e.g., after multiple transfusions)
    Irradiation
    Neoplasm
Pseudohypoparathyroidism (types I and II)
Hyperphosphatemia
  Phosphate administration
    Enemas, laxatives
    Intravenous administration
    Cow's milk in infant formula
  Renal failure (chronic or acute)
  Rhabdomyolysis
  Cytotoxic therapy for leukemia, lymphoma
Malignancy
  Osteoblastic metastases (especially carcinoma of prostate, breast)
  Malignancy with increased thyrocalcitonin levels (especially medullary carcinoma of thyroid)
Magnesium depletion (see 1-Q)
Drugs
  Loop diuretics
  Agents causing decreased bone resorption (e.g., actinomycin, calcitonin, mithramycin)
  Calcium-complexing agents (e.g., citrate, EDTA)
Massive transfusion, plasma exchange

Acute pancreatitis
Healing phase of rickets, osteitis fibrosa, thyrotoxic osteopathy ("hungry bone syndrome")
Hyperkalemic periodic paralysis, acute
Osteopetrosis
Neonatal tetany

References

1. Benabe JE, Martinez-Maldonado M: Disorders of Calcium Metabolism. In general reference 6, p 759.
2. Popovtzer MM, Knochel JP, Kumar R: Disorders of Calcium, Phosphorus, Vitamin D, and Parathyroid Hormone Activity. In general reference 16, p 287.

*Normal serum ionized calcium.

1-N. Hyperphosphatemia

Decreased Excretion and/or Increased Load
Renal failure (acute or chronic)
Oral or intravenous phosphate
Phosphate-containing laxatives, enemas
Transfusion of stored blood
Acidosis (especially lactic acidosis or diabetic ketoacidosis)
Rhabdomyolysis
Cytotoxic therapy for malignancy
Hemolysis, resolving hematoma
Increased intestinal absorption (e.g., vitamin D intoxication)
Malignant hyperpyrexia
Phosphorus burns
Familial (rare)

Increased Renal Tubular Reabsorption
Hypoparathyroidism
Pseudohypoparathyroidism
Hyperthyroidism
Volume contraction
High atmospheric temperature
Postmenopausal state
Diphosphonate therapy
Acromegaly
Juvenile hypogonadism
Tumoral calcinosis

Reference

1. Brautbar N, Kleeman CR: Hypophosphatemia and Hyperphosphatemia: Clinical and Pathophysiologic Aspects. In general reference 6, p 789.

1-O. Hypophosphatemia

Decreased Intake and Absorption and/or Increased Nonrenal Loss

Phosphate-binding antacids
Starvation, cachexia
Vomiting
Diarrhea, malabsorption
Hemodialysis

Transcellular Shift

Glucose infusion (with or without insulin administration)
Nutritional recovery syndrome
Alkalosis, respiratory
Androgens, anabolic steroids
Catecholamines (excessive secretion)
Infusion of:
   Bicarbonate
   Lactate
   Glucagon
Sepsis (especially gram-negative)
Thyrotoxicosis
Heat stroke
Gout, acute
Salicylate poisoning
Pregnancy
Myocardial infarction, acute

Renal Loss

Hyperparathyroidism, primary
Diuretic therapy
Volume expansion (including hyperaldosteronism)
Hypokalemia
Hypomagnesemia
Steroid therapy, Cushing's syndrome
Estrogens, oral contraceptives
Acidosis (especially metabolic)
Renal transplantation

Renal tubular defects (e.g., Fanconi's syndrome, vitamin D–resistant rickets)
Tumor phosphaturia (mesenchymoma, neurofibroma, pleomorphic sarcoma, sclerosing or cavernous hemangioma)

Multiple Mechanisms
Alcoholism and alcoholic withdrawal
Diabetic ketoacidosis
Liver disease, hepatic coma
Hyperalimentation
Vitamin D deficiency
Recovery from severe burns

References
1. Brautbar N, Kleeman CR: Hypophosphatemia and Hyperphosphatemia: Clinical and Pathophysiologic Aspects. In general reference 6, p 789.
2. Popovtzer MM, Knochel JP, Kumar R: Disorders of Calcium, Phosphorus, Vitamin D, and Parathyroid Hormone Activity. In general reference 16, p 287.

1-P. Hypermagnesemia

Renal failure, acute and chronic
Increased magnesium load (especially in presence of renal insufficiency)
    Magnesium-containing laxatives, antacids, or enemas
    Treatment of eclampsia (mother and infant)
    Diabetic ketoacidosis
Increased renal magnesium reabsorption
    Hyperparathyroidism
    Familial hypocalciuric hypercalcemia
    Hypothyroidism
    Mineralocorticoid deficiency, adrenal insufficiency

References
1. Brautbar N, Massry SG: Hypomagnesemia and Hypermagnesemia. In general reference 6, p 831.
2. Alfrey AC: Normal and Abnormal Magnesium Metabolism. In general reference 16, p 371.

1-Q. Hypomagnesemia

Redistribution
Postparathyroidectomy
Correction of metabolic acidosis (especially diabetic ketoacidosis)
Intravenous glucose, hyperalimentation
Refeeding after starvation
Acute pancreatitis

Decreased Intake and/or Increased Extrarenal Loss
Alcoholism
Malnutrition, poor intake
Nasogastric suction
Diarrhea, malabsorption (especially involving distal ileum)
Small bowel resection
Intestinal or biliary fistula
Profuse sweating, burns
Lactation

Increased Renal Loss
Drugs
  Diuretics
  Aminoglycosides
  Cisplatin
  Amphotericin B
Alcohol abuse
Diabetic ketoacidosis
Saline or osmotic diuresis
Postobstructive or postacute renal failure diuresis
Tubulointerstitial renal disease
Hypercalcemic states
Primary or secondary aldosteronism
Potassium depletion
Hypoparathyroidism
Hyperthyroidism
Syndrome of inappropriate antidiuretic hormone secretion
Familial

References
1. Brautbar N, Massry SG: Hypomagnesemia and Hypermagnesemia. In general reference 6, p 831.
2. Alfrey AC: Normal and Abnormal Magnesium Metabolism. In general reference 16, p 371.

2 CARDIOVASCULAR SYSTEM

2-A. Chest Pain

Skin and subcutaneous lesions (including adiposis dolorosa, thrombophlebitis of thoracoepigastric vein [Mondor's disease])
Breast lesions
  Fibroadenosis
  Chronic cystic mastitis
  Acute breast abscess or mastitis
  Carcinoma
Musculoskeletal disorders
  Bruised or fractured rib
  Periostitis
  Periosteal hematoma
  Costochondritis (Tietze's syndrome)
  Slipping costal cartilage
  Intercostal muscle "stitch" or cramp
  Intercostal myositis
  Pectoral or other muscular strain
  Shoulder girdle disorders (e.g., subacromial bursitis)
  Cervical disk herniation

    Dorsal spine osteoarthritis
    Thoracic outlet syndrome
Neuralgia
    Herpes zoster
    Tabes dorsalis
    Neurofibroma
    Neoplasm
Pericardial disease
    Pericarditis (see 2-I)
    Neoplasm
    Congenital absence of left pericardium
Mediastinal disease
    Mediastinal emphysema
    Neoplasm
    Mediastinitis
Cardiovascular disease
    Acute myocardial infarction
    Angina pectoris
    Aortic valvular disease
    Hypertrophic cardiomyopathy
    Mitral valve prolapse
    Acute aortic dissection
    Thoracic aortic aneurysm
    Myocarditis
    Primary pulmonary hypertension
    Ruptured sinus of Valsalva aneurysm
Pleural or pulmonary disease
    Pleuritis of any etiology (e.g., pneumothorax; see 13-F)
    Tracheobronchitis
    Pneumonia
    Pulmonary hypertension (see 13-O)
    Pulmonary thromboembolism
    Neoplasm
        Bronchogenic carcinoma
        Metastatic tumor
        Mesothelioma
    Other parenchymal lesions
Gastrointestinal disease
    Esophageal lesions
        Esophagitis
        Esophageal spasm
        Mallory-Weiss syndrome
        Esophageal rupture
        Foreign body
        Carcinoma
        Zenker's diverticulum
        Plummer-Vinson syndrome

Peptic ulcer disease (with or without perforation)
Gastric distention
Biliary disease
    Acute cholecystitis
    Biliary colic
Distention of the liver
Pancreatitis
Subphrenic abscess
Splenic infarct
Splenic flexure syndrome
Thyroiditis
Psychogenic causes

References
1. General reference 4, p 227.
2. Goldman L, Braunwald E: Chest Discomfort and Palpitation. In general reference 1, p 98.
3. Braunwald E: The History. In general reference 7, p 4.

2-B. Edema

Localized
Venous or lymphatic obstruction and/or insufficiency
    Venous thrombosis
    Baker's cyst
    Tumor invasion or compression (e.g., superior vena cava
        syndrome)
    Surgical or radiation damage
    Filariasis
Inflammatory disease
Allergic process
Physical or chemical trauma
Stings and bites
Immobilized or paralyzed limb
Congenital lymphedema

Generalized
Biventricular congestive heart failure (see 2-G)
Tricuspid stenosis
Cor pulmonale (see 13-O)
Pericardial disease (see 2-I, 2-J)
    Chronic constrictive pericarditis
    Pericardial effusion

Hypoalbuminemic states
    Hepatic cirrhosis
    Nephrotic syndrome
    Protein-losing enteropathy
    Malnutrition
    Severe chronic disease
Acute and chronic renal failure with volume overload
Inferior vena cava obstruction
Myxedema
Pregnancy
Iatrogenic salt overload
    Enteral feeding
    Intravenous fluid administration
    Drugs
        Carbenicillin and similar drugs
        Tamoxifen
        Estrogens
        Corticosteroids
        Minoxidil
        Calcium channel blockers (e.g., nifedipine)
        Guanethidine
        Diazoxide
Trichinosis
Idiopathic cyclic edema
Hereditary angioneurotic edema

Reference
1. Braunwald E: Edema. In general reference 1, p 228.

2-C. Palpitation*

Palpitation Without Arrhythmia
Noncardiac disorders
    Anxiety
    Exercise
    Anemia
    Fever
    Volume depletion
    Postural hypotension
    Thyrotoxicosis
    Menopausal syndrome
    Hypoglycemia

    Pheochromocytoma
    Aortic aneurysm
    Migraine syndrome
    Arteriovenous fistula
    Diaphragmatic flutter
    Drugs
        Sympathomimetic agents
        Ganglionic blockers
        Digitalis
        Nitrates
        Aminophylline
        Atropine
        Coffee, tea
        Tobacco
        Alcohol
        Thyroid extract
Cardiac disorders
    Aortic regurgitation
    Aortic stenosis
    Patent ductus arteriosus
    Ventricular septal defect
    Atrial septal defect
    Marked cardiomegaly
    Acute left ventricular failure
    Hyperkinetic heart syndrome
    Tricuspid insufficiency
    Pericarditis
    Prosthetic heart valve
    Electronic pacemaker

Palpitation with Arrhythmia†
Extrasystoles
Bradyarrhythmias
Tachyarrhythmias

Reference
1. Goldman L, Braunwald E: Chest Discomfort and Palpitation. In general reference 1, p 103.

*Palpitation is the sensation of disturbed heartbeat. This entry was modified from Shander D: Palpitation and Disorders of Heartbeat. In Friedman HH (ed): *Problem-Oriented Medical Diagnosis* (5th ed). Boston: Little, Brown, 1991, p 117.
†See 2-O.

2-D. Hypertension*

Systolic and Diastolic
Pseudohypertension (e.g., wrong-sized cuff)
Primary (essential)
Renal causes
   Parenchymal
   Vascular
   Renoprival (following bilateral nephrectomy)
   Renin-producing tumor
   Liddle's syndrome
Endocrine causes
   Acromegaly
   Hypothyroidism
   Hypercalcemia
   Adrenal causes
      Congenital adrenal hyperplasia
      Cushing's syndrome
      Primary aldosteronism
      Pheochromocytoma
   Extraadrenal chromaffin tumors
   Exogenous
      Oral contraceptives
      Estrogens
      Glucocorticoids
      Mineralocorticoids (e.g., licorice)
      Sympathomimetic agents
      Tyramine-containing foods and monoamine oxidase inhibitors
Coarctation of aorta
Pregnancy-induced
Neurogenic causes
   Increased intracranial pressure
   Postoperative state
   Acute porphyria
   Lead poisoning
   Quadriplegia (acute)
   Diencephalic syndrome
   Familial dysautonomia
Increased intravascular volume
   Polycythemia vera
   Iatrogenic causes
Burns
Sleep apnea
Psychogenic causes
Drug withdrawal

Other drugs
  Cocaine
  Cyclosporine
  Erythropoietin

Systolic
Increased cardiac output and/or stroke volume
  Aortic valvular regurgitation
  Fever
  Arteriovenous fistula, patent ductus arteriosus
  Paget's disease
  Beriberi
  Thyrotoxicosis (endogenous or exogenous)
  Anemia
  Hyperkinetic circulation
  Anxiety
  Complete heart block
Aortic rigidity

References
1. Kaplan NM: Systemic Hypertension: Mechanisms and Diagnosis. In general reference 7, p 817.
2. Williams GH, Braunwald E: Hypertensive Vascular Disease. In general reference 1, p 1001.

*Modified from Kaplan NM: Systemic Hypertension: Mechanisms and Diagnosis. In general reference 7, p 820.

2-E. Jugular Venous Distention

Extrathoracic Causes
Local venous obstruction of any cause (e.g., cervical goiter)
Circulatory overload of noncardiac etiology

Intrathoracic Causes
Valsalva maneuver
Retrosternal goiter
Superior vena cava syndrome
  Benign
  Malignant
Pericardial disease (see 2-I, 2-J)
  Cardiac tamponade
  Constrictive pericarditis

Cardiac disease
    Right heart failure of any etiology (e.g., tricuspid valve
        disease; see 2-G)
    Restrictive cardiomyopathy
    Right atrial myxoma
    Hyperkinetic heart circulatory states
Pleuropulmonary disease
    Pulmonary hypertension of any etiology (see 13-O)
    Bronchial asthma
    Chronic bronchitis and emphysema
    Tension pneumothorax

References

1. General reference 4, p 409.
2. Friedman HH: Jugular Venous Pulse. In general reference 3, p 9.

2-F. Heart Murmurs*

Systolic

Early systolic
    Physiologic (innocent)
    Small ventricular septal defect
    Large ventricular septal defect with pulmonary hyperten-
        sion
    Severe acute mitral or tricuspid regurgitation
    Tricuspid regurgitation without pulmonary hypertension
Midsystolic
    Physiologic (innocent)
        Vibratory murmur
        Hyperkinetic states
        Pulmonary ejection murmur
        Aortic ejection murmur of old age
    Obstruction to left ventricular outflow
        Valvular aortic stenosis
        Supravalvular aortic stenosis
        Hypertrophic cardiomyopathy
        Aortic valve prosthesis
    Aortic dilatation
    Murmurs of mitral regurgitation (occasionally)
    Aortic flow murmur in aortic regurgitation
    Coarctation of aorta
    Supraclavicular arterial bruit
    Obstruction to right ventricular outflow
        Supravalvular pulmonary arterial stenosis

      Pulmonic valvular stenosis
      Subpulmonic (infundibular) stenosis
   Flow murmur of atrial septal defect
   Idiopathic dilatation of pulmonary artery
   Pulmonary hypertension of any cause (occasionally)
Late systolic
   Mitral valve prolapse
   Tricuspid valve prolapse
Holosystolic
   Mitral regurgitation
   Tricuspid regurgitation secondary to pulmonary hypertension
   Ventricular septal defect
   Patent ductus arteriosus or aorticopulmonary window with pulmonary hypertension

Diastolic
Early diastolic
   Aortic regurgitation
   Pulmonic regurgitation associated with pulmonary hypertension, congenital or valvular disease
Middiastolic
   Mitral stenosis
   Mitral valve prosthesis
   Tricuspid stenosis
   Atrial myxoma
   Left atrial ball-valve thrombus
   Austin Flint murmur
   Increased diastolic atrioventricular flow
      Hyperkinetic states
      Mitral and tricuspid regurgitation
      Left-to-right shunt (e.g., ventricular septal defect)
      Acute rheumatic valvulitis
      Complete heart block
   Coronary artery stenosis
Presystolic
   Mitral stenosis
   Tricuspid stenosis
   Atrial myxoma
   Left-to-right shunt
   Complete heart block
   Severe pulmonic stenosis
   Fourth heart sound
   Severe aortic insufficiency

Continuous
Pseudomurmur (e.g., pericardial friction rub)
Traumatic or surgical arteriovenous fistula

Patent ductus arteriosus
Surgically created aorticopulmonary fistula
Pulmonary arteriovenous fistula
Aorticopulmonary window without severe pulmonary hyper-
  tension
Pulmonary embolism
Coronary arteriovenous fistula
Ruptured sinus of Valsalva aneurysm
Coarctation of aorta
Bronchial artery collateral circulation
Lutembacher's syndrome
Anomalous left coronary artery
Intercostal arteriovenous fistula
Cervical venous hum
Mammary souffle
Aortic arch syndrome
Pulmonary artery branch stenosis or partial occlusion

References
1. Craige E, Braunwald E: The Physical Examination. In
   general reference 7, p 13.
2. O'Rourke RA, Braunwald E: Physical Examination of the
   Heart. In general reference 1, p 843.
3. Friedman HH: Cardiovascular Problems: Heart Murmurs.
   In general reference 3, p 75.

*See also 2-N.

2-G. Congestive Heart Failure

Left Heart Failure
Hypertensive heart disease
Coronary artery disease
Left ventricular diastolic dysfunction
Acute myocardial infarction
Aortic and mitral valvular disease
Cardiomyopathy (see 2-H)
Pericardial disease (see 2-I, 2-J)
Arrhythmias
Congenital heart disease
Endocarditis
Cardiotoxic drugs (e.g., Adriamycin)
Myocarditis
Acute rheumatic fever

Traumatic heart disease
Thyrotoxicosis
Thiamine deficiency
Anemia
Arteriovenous fistula (e.g., Paget's disease)
Neoplastic heart disease
Toxic shock syndrome
Pulmonary thromboembolism
Postcardioversion
Pregnancy
Left atrial thrombus

Right Heart Failure*
Associated with pulmonary venous hypertension (postcapillary)
  Cardiac disease (see Left Heart Failure)
  Pulmonary venous disease
    Mediastinal neoplasm or granuloma
    Mediastinitis and fibrosis
    Anomalous pulmonary venous return
    Congenital pulmonary venous stenosis
    Idiopathic pulmonary venoocclusive disease
Associated with pulmonary arterial hypertension (precapillary)
  Lung and pleural disease
    Chronic bronchitis, emphysema, and asthma
    Granulomatous disease (e.g., sarcoidosis)
    Pneumonia
    Fibrotic disease
    Neoplasm
    Chronic suppurative disease (e.g., bronchiectasis)
    Cystic fibrosis
    Collagen-vascular disease
    Other restrictive processes (see 13-N)
    Following lung resection
    Bronchopulmonary dysplasia
    Fibrothorax
  Chest wall deformity
    Kyphoscoliosis
    Thoracoplasty
  Congenital pulmonary hypoplasia (Down's syndrome)
  Alveolar hypoventilation
    Neuromuscular
    Primary alveolar hypoventilation
    Obesity
    Sleep apnea syndrome
  High-altitude pulmonary hypertension

Intracardiac disease
   Increased flow associated with large left-to-right shunt
      Patent ductus arteriosus
      Atrial septal defect
      Ventricular septal defect
      Sinus of Valsalva aneurysm
   Decreased flow
      Tetralogy of Fallot
      Peripheral pulmonary artery stenosis (or stenoses)
      Unilateral absence or stenosis of pulmonary artery
Vascular disease
   Pulmonary thromboembolic disease
      Thrombotic
      Septic
      Fat
      Air
      Amniotic fluid, trophoblastic
      Foreign material (e.g., talc)
      Parasitic
      Metastatic neoplasm
      Thrombosis associated with SS and SC hemoglobin
      Thrombosis associated with eclampsia
   Primary pulmonary hypertension
   Hepatic cirrhosis and/or partial thrombosis
   Chemically induced (e.g., aminorex)
   Persistent fetal circulation
   Pulmonary arteritis
      Polyarteritis nodosa
      Overlap vasculitis
      Churg-Strauss syndrome
      Behçet's syndrome
      Raynaud's disease
      Scleroderma
      CRST syndrome
      Schistosomiasis
      Rheumatoid arthritis
      Systemic lupus erythematosus
      Polymyositis, dermatomyositis
      Granulomatous arteritis (e.g., Wegener's granuloma-
         tosis)
      Takayasu's disease
      Hughes-Stovin syndrome
      Ankylosing spondylitis
      Ulcerative colitis
      Sarcoidosis
      Immunoblastic lymphadenopathy
      Eosinophilic pneumonias
      Cryoglobulinemia

Disseminated leukocytoclastic vasculitis
Hypersensitivity pneumonitis
Peripheral pulmonary artery stenosis
Unilateral stenosis or absence of pulmonary artery
Without pulmonary hypertension
Pulmonic stenosis
Tricuspid stenosis (nonrheumatic)
Tricuspid regurgitation not associated with pulmonary hypertension
Decreased right ventricular compliance
Ebstein's anomaly
Atrial myxoma

References

1. General reference 24, p 1823.
2. Grossman W, Braunwald E: Pulmonary Hypertension. In general reference 7, p 790.

*See 13-O.

2-H. Cardiomyopathy*

Dilated (formerly congestive)

Congenital
  Diabetes
  Familial
  Duchenne's muscular dystrophy
  Facioscapulohumeral muscular dystrophy
  Limb-girdle muscular dystrophy
  Myotonic dystrophy
  Refsum disease
  Glycogen storage disorders
  Mucopolysaccharidosis
  Fabry's disease
  Gaucher's disease
  Sphingolipidosis
Acquired
  Idiopathic
  Inflammatory
    Infective myocarditis
    Acquired immunodeficiency syndrome
    Noninfective
      Collagen diseases
      Granulomatous disease

Metabolic
  Hypoxia
  Nutritional
    Thiamine deficiency
    Kwashiorkor
    Pellagra
    Scurvy
    Hypervitaminosis D
    Obesity
    Selenium deficiency
    Carnitine deficiency
  Endocrine
    Acromegaly
    Thyrotoxicosis
    Myxedema
    Uremia
    Cushing's disease
    Pheochromocytoma
    Diabetes
    Hypophosphatemia
    Hypocalcemia
  Altered metabolism
    Gout
    Porphyria
    Oxalosis
  Electrolyte imbalance
Toxins, drugs
  Disopyramide
  Daunorubicin
  Doxorubicin (Adriamycin)
  Cyclophosphamide
  Cocaine
  Bleomycin
  5-Fluorouracil
  Phosphate (poisoning)
  Phenothiazines and antidepressants
  Lithium
  Carbon monoxide
  Emetine
  Chloroquine
  Acetaminophen, paracetamol
  Lead
  Arsenic
  Hydrocarbons
  Antimony
  Cobalt
  Snake or insect bites
  Methysergide

Infiltrative
  Collagen vascular disease
  Amyloidosis
  Hemochromatosis
  Neoplastic
  Sarcoidosis
  Whipple's disease
Hematologic
  Leukemia
  Thrombotic thrombocytopenic purpura
  Sickle cell anemia
  Polycythemia vera
Hypersensitivity
  Methyldopa
  Penicillin
  Sulfonamides
  Tetracycline
  Phenindione
  Antituberculous drugs
  Giant cell myocarditis
  Cardiac transplant rejection
Peripartum
Vasculitis
Physical agents
  Irradiation
  Trauma
  Heat stroke
  Hypothermia
  Chronic tachycardia

Restrictive
Pseudocardiomyopathy (i.e., constrictive pericarditis)
Amyloidosis
Hemochromatosis
Sarcoidosis
Neoplasm
Endocardial fibroelastosis
Löffler's fibroplastic endocarditis (hypereosinophilic syndrome)
Endomyocardial fibrosis
Carcinoid

Hypertrophic
Idiopathic hypertrophic cardiomyopathy
Idiopathic nonobstructive cardiomyopathy
Glycogen storage disease (Pompe's disease)
Friedreich's ataxia
Lentiginosis

References

1. Wynne J, Braunwald E: The Cardiomyopathies and Myo-carditides. In general reference 7, p 1394.
2. Goodwin JF: Congestive and Hypertrophic Cardiomyopathies: A Decade of Study. *Lancet* 1:731, 1970.

---

*The distinction between cardiomyopathy by functional impairment is not absolute and overlap occurs frequently.

2-I. Pericarditis*

Idiopathic†
Infection
    Viral (e.g., acquired immunodeficiency syndrome
        [AIDS])†
    Bacterial†
    Mycobacterial†
    Mycoplasmal
    Fungal†
    Parasitic†
    Spirochetal (e.g., Lyme disease)
Acute myocardial infarction
Uremia†
Neoplasm†
Aortic dissection with hemopericardium
Connective-tissue or hypersensitivity diseases†
    Post–myocardial infarction (Dressler's syndrome)
    Postpericardiectomy
    Drugs
        Penicillin
        Isoniazid
        Methysergide
        Daunorubicin and doxorubicin
        Emetine
        Cromolyn (rare)
        Minoxidil
        Dantrolene
        Bleomycin
        Cyclophosphamide
        Practolol
    Systemic lupus erythematosus
        Idiopathic
        Drug-related
            Hydralazine
            Procainamide

      Phenytoin
      Isoniazid
      Methyldopa
   Mixed connective-tissue disease
   Scleroderma
   Wegener's granulomatosis
   Rheumatoid arthritis
   Polyarteritis nodosa
   Polymyositis
   Reiter's syndrome
   Ankylosing spondylitis
   Serum sickness
   Acute rheumatic fever
Trauma†
   Penetrating wounds
   Catheter- or pacemaker-induced cardiac perforation
   Blunt chest trauma
   Cardiopulmonary resuscitation
   Cardiothoracic surgery
   Cardioversion
   Pancreatic-pericardial fistula
Chylopericardium
Pseudoaneurysm Neptune
Cholesterol pericarditis
   Idiopathic
   Rheumatoid arthritis
   Hypercholesterolemia
   Myxedema
   Tuberculosis
Talc or other foreign substance
Sarcoidosis
Postirradiation†
Esophageal rupture
Uncommon miscellaneous etiologies
   Congenital heart disease (e.g., atrial septal defect)
   Familial Mediterranean fever
   Right atrial myxoma
   Degos' disease
   Gaucher's disease
   Myeloid metaplasia
   Amyloidosis
   Silicosis
   Giant cell arteritis
   Scorpion fish sting
   Pseudomyxoma peritonei
   Severe chronic anemia (e.g., thalassemia)
   Pancreatitis
   Whipple's disease

Acute gouty arthritis
Associated with atrial septal defect
Pulmonary thromboembolism
Takayasu's disease
Mulibrey nanism†
Nontraumatic hemopericardium
Inflammatory bowel disease
Behçet's disease

References

1. Lorell BH, Braunwald E: Pericardial Disease. In general reference 7, p 1465.
2. Braunwald E: Pericardial Disease. In general reference 1, p 981.

*See also 2-J.
†May be commonly associated with development of constrictive pericarditis.

2-J. Pericardial Effusion

Pericarditis of any cause (see 2-I)*
Congestive heart failure
Hypoalbuminemia
Acute pancreatitis
Chylopericardium*
   Congenital, idiopathic
   Neoplasm (e.g., lymphoma)
   After cardiothoracic surgery
   Benign obstruction of thoracic duct
Hemopericardium†
   Trauma
      Blunt and/or penetrating
      Iatrogenic
   Anticoagulants
   Chemotherapeutic agents
   Myocardial infarction
   Cardiac rupture
   Aortic or pulmonary artery rupture
   Coagulopathy
   Uremia
Myxedema*

References
1. Lorell BH, Braunwald E: Pericardial Disease. In general reference 7, p 1465.
2. Roberts WC, Spray TL: Pericardial Heart Disease. *Curr Prob Cardiol* 2(3):55, 1977.

*May be associated with chronic constrictive pericarditis.
†May be associated with acute cardiac tamponade.

2-K. Hypotension and Shock

Hypovolemia
  External losses
    Hemorrhage
    Gastrointestinal loss
    Renal loss
      Diuretics
      Diabetes insipidus
      Osmotic diuresis (e.g., diabetes mellitus)
      Diuretic phase of acute renal failure
      Salt-losing nephropathy
      Postobstructive diuresis
    Cutaneous loss
      Burns
      Exudative lesions
      Perspiration and insensible loss without replacement
  Internal losses
    Hemorrhage (e.g., anticoagulant therapy)
      Hemothorax
      Hemoperitoneum
      Retroperitoneal hemorrhage
      Soft tissue injury
      Fracture
    Fluid sequestration
      Ascites
      Bowel obstruction or infarction
      Peritonitis
      Phlegmon (e.g., pancreatitis)
Cardiovascular causes
  Arrhythmia (see 2-O)
  Regurgitant lesions
    Acute mitral or aortic regurgitation
    Rupture of interventricular septum
    Giant left ventricular aneurysm

Obstructive lesions
    Valvular stenosis
    Hypertrophic cardiomyopathy
    Atrial myxoma
    Intracardiac or valvular thrombus
Myopathy
    Acute myocardial infarction
    Dilated or restrictive cardiomyopathy (see 2-H)
    Other myocardial disorders (associated with low cardiac output)
Pericardial disease (see 2-I, 2-J)
    Cardiac tamponade
    Constrictive pericarditis
Aortic lesions
    Acute dissection
    Coarctation
    Rupture (e.g., trauma or aneurysm)
Congenital heart disease
Vena cava obstruction
Pleuropulmonary disease
    Tension pneumothorax
    Positive pressure ventilation
    Pulmonary embolism (including thrombus, amniotic fluid, air, tumor)
    Primary or secondary pulmonary hypertension
    Eisenmenger reaction
Infection
    Septicemia
    Specific infections (e.g., dengue fever)
    Toxic shock syndrome
Anaphylaxis
Endocrine disease
    Adrenal insufficiency
    Hypoglycemia or hyperglycemia
    Hypocalcemia or hypercalcemia
    Myxedema or thyroid storm
    Pheochromocytoma
    Pituitary failure including diabetes insipidus
Hypoxia
Severe acidosis or alkalosis
Nonbacterial sepsis syndrome
Hypothermia or hyperthermia
Hepatic failure
Drugs and toxins
    Drug overdose and poisoning (e.g., barbiturates)
    Antihypertensive agents
    Other vasodilators (e.g., nitroglycerin)
    Heavy metals

Hyperviscosity syndrome
Neuropathic causes
   Brainstem failure
   Spinal cord dysfunction
   Autonomic insufficiency

References
1. Parrillo JE: Shock. In general reference 1, p 232.
2. Weil MH, Planta MV, Rackow EC: Acute Circulatory Failure (Shock). In general reference 7, p 569.

2-L. Cardiac Arrest (Sudden Cardiopulmonary Collapse)

Arrhythmia (with or without digitalis intoxication)
   Tachyarrhythmia
      Ventricular fibrillation (e.g., prolonged QT syndromes)
      Ventricular tachycardia
   Bradyarrhythmia
      Sinus bradycardia
      Junctional rhythm
      Atrioventricular block
      Idioventricular rhythm
   Asystole
Upper airway obstruction
   Structural lesion
   Sleep apnea syndrome
   Foreign body
Acute and/or chronic respiratory failure with hypoxemia
      and/or hypercarbia
Hypoxia of any cause (e.g., carbon monoxide poisoning)
Pulmonary hypertension
Smoke inhalation
Severe acidosis or alkalosis
Hypoglycemia
Syncope (see 12-D)
Addisonian crisis
Drug overdose, allergy, or adverse reaction
   Narcotics
   Insulin
   Sedatives
   Digitalis
   Quinidine
   Cocaine
   Disopyramide

Procainamide and other antiarrhythmics
Phenothiazines
Tricyclic antidepressants
Nitrates
Aminophylline
Propranolol
Warfarin
Penicillins
Sulfonamides
Antihypertensive agents
Shock of any etiology (see also 2-K), especially:
Hypovolemia
Tension pneumothorax
Cardiac tamponade or pericardial constriction
Anaphylaxis
Sepsis
Aortic dissection or rupture
Pulmonary embolism (of any type)
Acute myocardial infarction
Other common cardiac causes
Severe coronary heart disease
Valvular disease (e.g., aortic stenosis; see 2-N)
Prosthetic valve dysfunction
Myocarditis and cardiomyopathy (see 2-H)
Cardiac rupture
Congenital heart disease
Mitral valve prolapse
Primary conduction system or nodal disease
Nonatherosclerotic obstruction of coronary arteries
Embolus
Arteritis
Dissection (e.g., in pregnancy, Marfan's)
Spasm
Congenital anomalies
Coronary artery ostia obstruction (e.g., syphilis)
Electrolyte abnormality (especially potassium, calcium,
magnesium)
Hypothermia or hyperthermia
Electric shock
Drowning
Insect stings and bites
Neurologic disorders
Stroke
Hemorrhage
Seizure
Brainstem compression of any cause
Infection

Sudden infant death syndrome
Liquid protein diet
Modified fast diet programs

References
1. Myerburg RJ, Castellanos A: Cardiovascular Arrest and
   Sudden Cardiac Death. In general reference 7, p 756.
2. Myerburg RJ, Castellanos A: Cardiovascular Collapse,
   Cardiac Arrest, and Sudden Death. In general reference
   1, p 237.

2-M. Complications of Cardiopulmonary Resuscitation

Cerebral
  Hypoxic encephalopathy
Oronasopharyngeal
  Laceration
  Fractured teeth
  Epistaxis
  Laryngeal injury
Neck
  Spinal cord injury
  Vascular injury and hematoma
Lung and chest wall
  Pneumothorax and pneumomediastinum
  Subcutaneous emphysema
  Rib and sternal fractures
  Hemothorax
  Pulmonary contusion
  Atelectasis
    Malpositioned endotracheal tube
    Foreign body
    Secretions
  Aspiration
Heart and pericardium
  Hemopericardium and cardiac tamponade
  Lacerated heart or coronary vessels
  Ruptured ventricle
Visceral injury
  Acute gastric dilatation
  Gastroesophageal, liver, or splenic laceration
Acute renal failure
Fat embolism

Volume overload
Metabolic alkalosis
   Sodium bicarbonate administration
   Posthypercapnic
Bacteremia

Reference

1. Myerburg RJ, Castellanos A: Cardiovascular Arrest and Sudden Cardiac Death. In general reference 7, p 756.

2-N. Valvular Disease*

Aortic Valve
Stenosis
   Valvular
      Congenital
      Rheumatic
      Calcific (senile)
      Atherosclerotic
      Rheumatoid
      Ochronosis
   Supravalvular
   Subvalvular
Regurgitation
   Congenital
      Bicuspid aortic valve
         Isolated
         Associated with:
            Coarctation
            Ventricular septal defect
            Patent ductus arteriosus
      Tricuspid aortic valve
         Isolated
         Associated with:
            Ventricular septal defect
            Valvular aortic stenosis
            Supravalvular aortic stenosis
            Subvalvular aortic stenosis
            Congenital aneurysm of sinus of Valsalva
            Cusp fenestrations
      Quadricuspid aortic valve
   Acquired
      Valvular
         Rheumatic heart disease
         Bacterial endocarditis

Calcific aortic valve disease
Atherosclerosis
Traumatic valve rupture
Dissection of the aorta
Postaortic valve surgery
   Postvalvulotomy
   Leakage around prosthesis
   Endocarditis
Miscellaneous
   Ankylosing spondylitis
   Reiter's syndrome
   Rheumatoid arthritis
   Whipple's disease
   Crohn's disease
   Jaccoud's arthropathy
   Systemic lupus erythematosus
   Scleroderma
   Myxomatous degeneration
   Pseudoxanthoma elasticum
   Mucopolysaccharidoses
   Osteogenesis imperfecta
   Cusp fenestrations
   Methysergide
Aortic dilatation or distortion
   Senile dilatation
   Cystic medial necrosis with or without Marfan's syndrome
   Takayasu's disease
   Relapsing polychondritis
   Syphilis
   Ankylosing spondylitis
   Psoriatic arthritis
   Ulcerative colitis with arthritis
   Reiter's syndrome
   Giant cell arteritis
   Ehlers-Danlos syndrome
   Hypertension
   Cogan's syndrome
   Behçet's syndrome

Mitral Valve

Stenosis
   Congenital
   Rheumatic
   Carcinoid syndrome
   Marantic endocarditis
   Systemic lupus erythematosus
   Calcific

Lutembacher's syndrome
Amyloidosis
Rheumatoid arthritis
Hunter-Hurler disease
Methysergide
Regurgitation
  Congenital
    Isolated mitral regurgitation
    Idiopathic hypertrophic subaortic stenosis (IHSS)
    Connective-tissue disorders
      Ehlers-Danlos syndrome
      Hurler's syndrome
      Marfan's syndrome
      Pseudoxanthoma elasticum
      Osteogenesis imperfecta
    Atrioventricular cushion defect
    Endocardial fibroelastosis
    Parachute mitral valve complex
    Hypoplastic left heart syndrome
    Anomalous left coronary artery from pulmonary artery
    Congenital mitral stenosis
    Corrected transposition of great vessels with or without
        Ebstein's malformation
    Supravalvular ring of left atrium
  Acquired
    Coronary heart disease
    Rheumatic (acute or chronic)
    Mitral valve prolapse syndrome
    Papillary muscle dysfunction
      Coronary heart disease with or without myocardial
          infarction
      Neoplasm
      Myocardial abscess
      Granulomas
      Sarcoidosis
      Amyloidosis
    Ruptured or abnormal chordae tendineae (e.g., idio-
        pathic myxomatous proliferation)
    Bacterial endocarditis
    Calcified mitral annulus
      Idiopathic systemic hypertension
      Aortic stenosis
      Diabetes
      Chronic renal failure with secondary hyperparathy-
          roidism
    Left ventricular dilatation or aneurysm (e.g., dilated
        cardiomyopathy)
    Aortic valve disease

Prosthetic valve disruption
Trauma
Post–cardiac surgery
Rheumatoid arthritis
Ankylosing spondylitis
Scleroderma
Systemic lupus erythematosus
Left atrial myxoma
Spontaneous rupture
Carcinoid syndrome
Giant left atrium
Kawasaki disease
Hypereosinophilic syndrome

Pulmonic Valve
Stenosis
  Congenital
    Valvular stenosis
    Valvular dysplasia (e.g., Noonan's syndrome)
    Tetralogy of Fallot
    Supravalvular aortic stenosis syndrome
  Acquired
    Intrinsic valvular lesions
      Rheumatic disease
      Carcinoid syndrome
      Endocarditis
      Primary neoplasm
    Extrinsic lesions
      Neoplasm
      Aortic or septal aneurysm
      Sinus of Valsalva aneurysm
      Constrictive pericarditis
Regurgitation
  Congenital
    Absent pulmonic valve
    Isolated pulmonic regurgitation
    Associated with:
      Tetralogy of Fallot
      Ventricular septal defect
      Pulmonic valvular stenosis
      Idiopathic dilatation of pulmonic valve
  Acquired
    Valve ring dilatation secondary to pulmonary hypertension of any cause (see 2-G, Right Heart Failure)
    Pulmonary artery dilatation, idiopathic
    Bacterial endocarditis
    Post–pulmonic valve surgery
    Rheumatic disease

Trauma
Syphilis
Carcinoid syndrome
Marfan's syndrome
Induced by pulmonary artery catheter

Tricuspid Valve

Stenosis
  Rheumatic heart disease (acute and chronic)
  Carcinoid syndrome
  Fibroelastosis
  Tricuspid atresia
  Endomyocardial fibrosis
Regurgitation
  Right ventricular dilatation of any cause (e.g., mitral stenosis)
  Pulmonary hypertension (see 2-G, Right Heart Failure)
  Rheumatic heart disease
  Right ventricular papillary muscle dysfunction
  Myxomatous valve and chordae (usually in association with mitral valve prolapse with or without atrial septal defect)
  Trauma
  Bacterial endocarditis
  Carcinoid syndrome
  Ebstein's anomaly
  Common atrioventricular canal
  Ventricular septal aneurysm
  Right atrial myxoma
  Constrictive pericarditis
  Endomyocardial fibrosis
  Methysergide
  Systemic lupus erythematosus
  Radiation injury
  Thyrotoxicosis
  Isolated lesion
  Following surgical excision
  Marfan's syndrome
  Rheumatoid arthritis

References

1. Braunwald E: Valvular Heart Disease. In general reference 7, p 1007.
2. Braunwald E: Valvular Heart Disease. In general reference 1, p 938.

*See also 2-F.

2-O. Arrhythmias

Premature Beats
Extrasystole
  Sinus (rare)
  Atrial
  Atrioventricular junctional
  Ventricular
Parasystole
Capture beat
Reciprocal beat
Better atrioventricular conduction (e.g., 3 : 2), interrupting
    poorer (e.g., 2 : 1)
Supernormal conduction during advanced atrioventricular
    block
Rhythm resumption after inapparent bigeminy

Bradycardia (< 60 beats/min)
Sinus bradycardia
Atrioventricular junctional rhythm
Sinus arrhythmia
Wandering atrial pacemaker
Sinoatrial block (second and third degree)
Sinus pause or arrest
Nonconducted atrial or ventricular bigeminy
Hypersensitive carotid sinus syndrome
Atrioventricular block (second and third degree)
Supraventricular tachyarrhythmias with high-grade atrio-
    ventricular block (rare)
Escape rhythms (resulting from bradycardia of any cause)
  Atrioventricular junctional
  Idioventricular
Sick sinus syndrome

Tachycardia (Ventricular Rate > 100 Beats/Min)

	Rate		Carotid sinus massage
	Atrial	Ventricular	
NORMAL QRS (< 0.10 SEC)			
Regular Rhythm			
Sinus tachycardia	100–200 (usually < 160)	100–200 (usually < 160)	Gradual slowing with return to previous rate
Paroxysmal supraventricular tachycardia*	140–250	140–250	No effect or abrupt termination
Paroxysmal atrial tachycardia with block	140–250	Variable (usually 75–200)	May abruptly and transiently decrease ventricular rate; generally contraindicated
Atrial flutter	250–350	Variable (usually 75–175)	Transient slowing of ventricular rate, revealing flutter waves
Paroxysmal atrioventricular junctional tachycardia	140–250	140–250	No effect or abrupt termination
Nonparoxysmal atrioventricular junctional tachycardia	Depends on atrial mechanism	65–130	No effect or gradual slowing with return to previous rate; generally contraindicated

Irregular Rhythm

Atrial fibrillation*	350–600	Variable	Transient decrease in ventricular rate
Paroxysmal atrial tachycardia with variable block	140–250	Variable	May abruptly and transiently decrease ventricular rate; generally contraindicated
Atrial flutter with variable block	250–350	Variable	Transient slowing of ventricular rate, revealing flutter waves
Multifocal atrial tachycardia	100–200	100–200	No effect or gradual slowing

ABNORMAL QRS (> 0.10 SEC)

Regular Rhythm

Sinus tachycardia with preexisting bundle-branch block or preexcitation	100–200 (usually < 160)	100–200 (usually < 160)	Gradual slowing with return to previous rate
Paroxysmal supraventricular tachycardia with aberrant conduction, preexisting bundle-branch block, or preexcitation (rare)	140–250	140–250	No effect or abrupt termination

Tachycardia (Ventricular Rate > 100 Beats/Min) (continued)

	Rate		Carotid sinus massage
	Atrial	Ventricular	
ABNORMAL QRS (> 0.10 SEC)			
Regular Rhythm			
Paroxysmal supraventricular tachycardia with block, with aberrant conduction or preexisting bundle-branch block	140–250	Variable (usually < 170)	May abruptly and transiently decrease ventricular rate; generally contraindicated
Atrial flutter with aberrant conduction or preexisting bundle-branch block	250–350	Variable (usually 120–175)	Transient slowing of ventricular rate, revealing flutter waves
Atrioventricular junctional tachycardias with aberrant conduction or preexisting bundle-branch block			

Paroxysmal	140–250	140–250	No effect or abrupt termination
Nonparoxysmal	Depends on atrial mechanism	65–130	No effect or gradual slowing with return to previous rate; generally contraindicated
Ventricular tachycardia	Equal to or less than ventricular rate	60–250 (usually > 150 and may be slightly irregular)	Atrial rate may slow; no effect on ventricular rate
Irregular Rhythm			
Atrial fibrillation with aberrant conduction or preexisting bundle-branch block	350–600	Variable	Transient decrease in ventricular rate
Paroxysmal supraventricular tachycardia with variable block, with aberrant conduction, or preexisting bundle-branch block	140–250	Variable	May abruptly and transiently decrease ventricular rate; generally contraindicated

Tachycardia (Ventricular Rate > 100 Beats/Min) (continued)

	Rate		Carotid sinus massage
	Atrial	Ventricular	
ABNORMAL QRS (> 0.10 SEC)			
Irregular Rhythm			
Atrial flutter with variable block, with aberrant conduction or preexisting bundle-branch block	250–350	Variable	Transient slowing of ventricular rate, revealing flutter waves

*Arrhythmias most commonly associated with preexcitation (Wolff-Parkinson-White syndrome).
Source: Modified from Marriott HJL: *Practical Electrocardiography* (8th ed). Baltimore: Williams & Wilkins, 1988. Copyright © 1988 by The Williams & Wilkins Co., Baltimore.

References
1. Marriott HJL: *Practical Electrocardiography* (8th ed). Baltimore: Williams & Wilkins, 1988.
2. Friedman HH: *Diagnostic Electrocardiography and Vectorcardiography* (3rd ed). New York: McGraw-Hill, 1984.
3. Zipes, DP: Special Arrhythmias: Diagnosis and Treatment. In general reference 7, p 667.

2-P. Electrocardiographic Abnormalities

QRS Interval, Prolonged
Bundle-branch blocks
Nonspecific intraventricular conduction delay
Aberrant ventricular conduction
Ectopic ventricular rhythm (e.g., ventricular parasystole)
Drug effect (e.g., quinidine or procainamide)
Electrolyte abnormalities (hyperkalemia, hypokalemia, hypercalcemia, hypermagnesemia)
Preexcitation (Wolff-Parkinson-White syndrome)
Left ventricular enlargement
Periinfarction block
Hypothermia

ST Segment Changes
Elevation
   Normal variant (e.g., "early repolarization")
   Artifact
   Myocardial infarction
   Prinzmetal's angina
   Ventricular aneurysm
   Reciprocal changes
   Pericarditis
   Hyperkalemia (rarely)
   Bundle-branch block
   Acute cor pulmonale (e.g., pulmonary thromboembolism)
   Myocarditis
   Neoplastic heart disease
   Stroke
   Hypertrophic cardiomyopathy
   Hypothermia
Depression
   Nonspecific abnormality (e.g., anxiety, shock)
   Drugs
      Digitalis

    Tricyclic antidepressants
    Lithium
Bundle-branch block
Left or right ventricular strain
Electrolyte abnormalities (hyperkalemia or hypokalemia)
Subendocardial ischemia or infarction
Mitral valve prolapse
Tachycardia
Myocarditis or cardiomyopathy
Reciprocal changes
Cerebral or subarachnoid injury
Pancreatitis or other acute intraabdominal catastrophe
Pulmonary thromboembolism
Hypothyroidism

QT Interval

Prolonged
    Electrolyte abnormalities (hypocalcemia, hypokalemia,
      ["QU" prolongation])
    Complete heart block
    Mitral valve prolapse
    Left ventricular enlargement
    Myocardial infarction and ischemia
    Myocarditis and cardiomyopathy
    Diffuse myocardial disease
    Cerebral or subarachnoid injury, including surgical
    Drugs (e.g., quinidine, procainamide, phenothiazines,
      terfenadine)
    Hypothermia
    Heritable anomaly
    Alkalosis
Shortened
    Electrolyte abnormalities (hypercalcemia, hyperkalemia)
    Digitalis
    Acidosis

T-Wave Changes

Peaking
    Normal variant
    Nonspecific abnormality
    Electrolyte abnormalities (hyperkalemia, hypocalcemia,
      hypomagnesemia)
    Acute myocardial ischemia or infarction
    Reciprocal effect in strictly posterior myocardial infarction
    Left ventricular enlargement
    Anemia

Inversion
  Normal
  Juvenile T-wave pattern
  Left bundle-branch block
  Nonspecific abnormality
  Myocardial ischemia or infarction
  Myocarditis
  Pericarditis
  Ventricular strain
  Acute or chronic cor pulmonale
  Cerebral or subarachnoid injury
  Drugs (e.g., quinidine, phenothiazines)
  Electrolyte abnormalities (hypokalemia, hypocalcemia,
    hypomagnesemia)
  Complete atrioventricular block
  Vagotomy
  Following tachycardia

Q Waves, Abnormal
Myocardial infarction
Ischemia (transient)
Dextrocardia or dextroversion
Hypertrophic cardiomyopathy
Reversal of right and left arm leads (lead I)
Ventricular enlargement
Acute and chronic cor pulmonale (e.g., pulmonary embo-
  lism, chronic obstructive pulmonary disease)
Preexcitation
Cardiac surgery
Spontaneous pneumothorax (especially left)
Cardiomyopathy and myocarditis (e.g., hypertrophic cardio-
  myopathy; see 2-H)
Localized destructive myocardial disease (e.g., neoplasm)
Left bundle-branch block
Left anterior division block
Normal variant (rare)
Tachycardia (transitory)
Critical illness (e.g., pancreatitis, shock)

References
1. Friedman HH: *Diagnostic Electrocardiography and Vec-*
   torcardiography (3rd ed.) New York: McGraw-Hill, 1984.
2. Marriott HJL: *Practical Electrocardiography* (8th ed.)
   Baltimore: Williams & Wilkins, 1988.
3. Fisch C: Electrocardiography and Vectorcardiography. In
   general reference 7, p 116.

2-Q. Cardiac Risk Index for Noncardiac Surgical Procedures

Computation of the Cardiac Risk Index

Criteria	"Points"
1. History	
a. Age > 70 yr	5
b. MI in previous 6 mo	10
2. Physical examination	
a. S_3 gallop or JVD	11
b. Important VAS	3
3. Electrocardiogram	
a. Rhythm other than sinus or PACs on last preoperative ECG	7
b. > 5 PVCs/min documented at any time before operation	7
4. General status: PO_2 < 60 or PCO_2 > 50 mmHg, K < 3.0 or HCO_3^- < 20 mEq/L, BUN > 50 or Cr > 3.0 mg/dl, abnormal SGOT, signs of chronic liver disease, or patient bedridden from noncardiac causes	3
5. Operation	
a. Intraperitoneal, intrathoracic, or aortic	3
b. Emergency	4
Total possible:	53

MI = myocardial infarction; JVD = jugular vein distention; VAS = valvular aortic stenosis; PACs = premature atrial contractions; ECG = electrocardiogram; PVCs = premature ventricular contractions; PO_2 = partial pressure of oxygen; PCO_2 = partial pressure of carbon dioxide; K = potassium; HCO_3^- = bicarbonate; BUN = blood urea nitrogen; Cr = creatinine; and SGOT = serum glutamic oxaloacetic transaminase.

Source: Adapted from Goldman L, et al: Multifactorial Index of Cardiac Risk in Non-cardiac Surgical Procedures. *N Engl J Med* 297:848, 1977. By permission of the *New England Journal of Medicine*.

Cardiac Risk Index

Class	Point total	No (or only minor) complications (N = 943)	Life-threatening complication[a] (N = 39)	Cardiac deaths (N = 19)
I (N = 537)	0–5	532 (99)[b]	4 (0.7)	1 (0.2)
II (N = 316)	6–12	295 (93)	16 (5)	5 (2)
III (N = 130)	13–25	112 (86)	15 (11)	3 (2)
IV (N = 18)	> 26	4 (22)	4 (22)	10 (56)

[a] Documented intraoperative or postoperative myocardial infarction, pulmonary edema, or ventricular tachycardia without progression to cardiac death.

[b] Figures in parentheses denote percentages.

Source: Goldman L, et al: Multifactorial Index of Cardiac Risk in Non-cardiac Surgical Procedures. *N Engl J Med* 297:848, 1977. Reprinted by permission of the *New England Journal of Medicine*.

References
1. Goldman L, Braunwald E: General Anesthesia and Non-cardiac Surgery in Patients with Heart Disease. In general reference 7, p 1708.
2. Goldman L, et al: Multifactorial Index of Cardiac Risk in Non-cardiac Surgical Procedures. *N Engl J Med* 297:845, 1977.
3. Goldman L: Multifactoral Index of Cardiac Risk in Non-cardiac Surgery. Ten-year Status Report. *J Cardiothorac Anesth* 1:237, 1987
4. Gerson MC, et al: Prediction of Cardiac and Pulmonary Complications Related to Elective Abdominal and Non-cardiac Thoracic Surgery in Geriatric Patients. *Am J Med* 88:101, 1990

3 DRUGS

3-A. Bacterial Endocarditis Prophylaxis in Adults

CARDIAC CONDITIONS

Endocarditis Prophylaxis Recommended

Prosthetic cardiac valves (bioprosthetic and homograft valves)

Previous bacterial endocarditis (even without heart disease)

Congenital cardiac malformations (most)

Rheumatic and other acquired valvular dysfunction (even after valvular surgery)

Hypertrophic cardiomyopathy (idiopathic hypertrophic subaortic stenosis)

Mitral valve prolapse with valvular regurgitation

Endocarditis Prophylaxis Not Recommended

Isolated secundum atrial septal defect

Surgical repair without residua beyond 6 mo of secundum atrial septal defect, ventricular septal defect, patent ductus arteriosus

Previous coronary artery bypass graft surgery

Mitral valve prolapse without valvular regurgitation[a]
Physiologic, functional, or innocent heart murmurs
Previous Kawasaki's disease without valvular
dysfunction
Previous rheumatic fever without valvular dysfunction
Cardiac pacemakers and implanted defibrillators

DENTAL OR SURGICAL PROCEDURES

Endocarditis Prophylaxis Recommended

Dental procedures known to induce gingival or mucosal
bleeding, including professional cleaning
Tonsillectomy and/or adenoidectomy
Surgical operations involving intestinal or respiratory
mucosa
Bronchoscopy with a rigid bronchoscope
Sclerotherapy for esophageal varices
Esophageal dilatation
Gallbladder surgery
Cystoscopy
Urethral dilatation
Urethral catheterization, with urinary tract infection[b]
Urinary tract surgery, with urinary tract infection[b]
Prostatic surgery
Incision and drainage of infected tissue[b]
Vaginal hysterectomy
Vaginal delivery in the presence of infection[b]

Endocarditis Prophylaxis Not Recommended[c]

Dental procedures not likely to induce gingival bleeding
(e.g., simple adjustment of orthodontic appliances or
fillings above the gum line)
Injection of local intraoral anesthetic (except
intraligamentary injections)
Shedding of primary teeth
Tympanostomy tube insertion
Endotracheal intubation
Bronchoscopy (flexible bronchoscope, with or without
biopsy)
Cardiac catheterization
Endoscopy, with or without gastrointestinal biopsy
Cesarean section

In the absence of infection for urethral catheterization, dilatation and curettage, uncomplicated vaginal delivery, therapeutic abortion, sterilization procedures, or insertion or removal of intrauterine devices

---

[a] Patients with mitral valve prolapse associated with thickening and/or redundancy of the valve leaflets may be at increased risk for endocarditis, particularly if they are men over age 45.

[b] In addition to prophylactic regimen for genitourinary procedures, antibiotic therapy should be directed against the most likely bacterial pathogen.

[c] In patients with prosthetic heart valves or a previous history of endocarditis, physicians may elect prophylaxis even for low-risk procedures that involve the lower respiratory, genitourinary, or gastrointestinal tract.

Source: From Dajani AS, et al: Prevention of Bacterial Endocarditis. *JAMA* 264:2919, 1990.

Prophylactic Regimens

Procedure	Recommended treatment
DENTAL, ORAL, OR UPPER RESPIRATORY TRACT PROCEDURES IN PATIENTS AT RISK	
Standard	
For ampicillin-/amoxicillin-/penicillin-allergic patients	Amoxicillin, 3 gm PO 1 hr before procedure; then 1.5 gm PO 6 hr after initial dose
	Erythromycin ethylsuccinate, 800 mg PO, or erythromycin stearate, 1 gm PO, 2 hr before procedure; then erythromycin ethylsuccinate, 400 mg PO, or erythromycin stearate, 500 mg PO, 6 hr after initial administration
	or
	Clindamycin, 300 mg PO 1 hr before procedure; then 150 mg 6 hr after initial dose
Alternate	
For patients unable to take oral medication	Ampicillin, 2 gm IV (or IM) 30 min before procedure; then ampicillin, 1 gm IV (or IM), or amoxicillin, 1.5 gm PO, 6 hr after initial dose
For ampicillin-/amoxicillin-/penicillin-allergic patients unable to take oral medication	Clindamycin, 300 mg IV 30 min before procedure; then 150 mg IV (or PO) 6 hr after initial dose

For patients considered to be at very high risk

Ampicillin, 2 gm IV (or IM) plus gentamicin 1.5 mg/kg IV (or IM)—not to exceed 80 mg—30 min before procedure; then amoxicillin, 1.5 gm PO 6 hr after initial dose. Alternatively, parenteral regimen can be repeated 8 hr after initial dose*

For amoxicillin-/ampicillin-/penicillin-allergic patients considered to be at very high risk

Vancomycin, 1 gm IV administered over 1 hr, starting 1 hr before procedure; no repeat dose is necessary

FOR GENITOURINARY AND GASTROINTESTINAL PROCEDURES

Standard

Ampicillin, 2 gm IV (or IM) plus gentamicin 1.5 mg/kg IV (or IM)—not to exceed 80 mg—30 min before procedure; then amoxicillin, 1.5 gm PO 6 hr after initial dose. Alternatively, parenteral regimen can be repeated once 8 hr after initial dose*

For amoxicillin-/ampicillin-/penicillin-allergic patients

Vancomycin, 1 gm IV administered over 1 hr plus gentamicin, 1.5 mg/kg IV (or IM)—not to exceed 80 mg—1 hr before procedure. May be repeated once 8 hr after initial dose*

Alternate

For low-risk patients

Amoxicillin, 3 gm PO 1 hr before procedure; then 1.5 gm 6 hr after initial dose

Prophylactic Regimens (continued)

Procedure	Recommended treatment
FOR CARDIAC SURGERY WITH PLACEMENT OF FOREIGN MATERIAL	
Standard	Cefazolin, 2 gm IV plus gentamicin, 1.5 mg/kg IV immediately preoperatively and q8h for 24 hr*
Alternate	
In institutions with a high incidence of methicillin-resistant staphylococci	Vancomycin, 15 mg/kg IV administered over 1 hr immediately preoperatively; then vancomycin 10 mg/kg IV administered over 1 hr immediately after surgery plus gentamicin as specified above (see standard)

*Dose modification may be required in renal insufficiency.
Source: Modified from Dajani AS, et al: Prevention of Bacterial Endocarditis. *JAMA* 264:2919, 1990; and Korzeniowski OM, Kaye D: Infective Endocarditis. In general reference 7, p 1078.

References
1. Korzeniowski OM, Kaye D: Infective Endocarditis. In general reference 7, p 1078.
2. Dajani AS, et al: Prevention of Bacterial Endocarditis. *JAMA* 264:2919, 1990.

3-B. Isoniazid Prophylaxis of Tuberculous Infection*†

Eligible persons are listed by priority grouping:

1. Household members and others in close contact with an infectious case‡
2. Positive tuberculin reactors who have chest x-ray findings characteristic of inactive tuberculous infection with a life expectancy of greater than 10 years
3. Recent tuberculin skin-test converters (i.e., skin test induration has increased by at least 6 mm, from less than 10 mm to more than 10 mm in less than 24 mo)
4. Positive tuberculin reactors who have any of the following conditions:
   a. Chronic corticosteroid or immunosuppressive therapy
   b. Chronic malignancy, especially lymphoma or leukemia
   c. Silicosis
   d. Diabetes mellitus
   e. Malnutrition (especially postgastrectomy)
   f. Chronic renal failure
   g. Acquired immunodeficiency syndrome (AIDS)
5. Positive tuberculin reactors under age 20–35 who have never received isoniazid prophylaxis

References
1. Des Prez RM, Heim CR: Mycobacterium Tuberculosis. In Mandell GL, et al (eds): *Principles and Practice of Infectious Diseases* (3rd ed). New York: Churchill Livingstone, 1993, p 1877.
2. Jordan TJ, Lewitt EM, Reichman LB: Isoniazid Preventive Therapy for Tuberculosis. *Am Rev Respir Dis* 144:1357; 1991.

---

*Before isoniazid chemoprophylaxis is begun, it is essential to exclude active infection (for which single-drug therapy is inadequate).
†If isoniazid resistance is suspected, an alternative prophylactic regimen may be appropriate.
‡Treatment can be stopped if a patient's skin test is negative after 3 mos of therapy.

3-C. Guidelines For Tetanus Prophylaxis

History of Tetanus Immunization (doses)	Years since last dose	Clean minor wounds		All Other Wounds	
		Give Td[a]	Give TIG	Give Td	Give TIG[b]
Unknown or < 3	—	Yes	No	Yes	Yes[c]
≥ 3	> 10	Yes	No	Yes	No
≥ 3	5–10	No	No	Yes	No
≥ 3	< 5	No	No	No[d]	No

[a]Adult-type tetanus and diphtheria toxoids (Td) for patients > 6 yr old.
[b]Human tetanus immune globulin (TIG) is preferred given as 250 units IM.
[c]500 units IM is preferred for highly tetanus-prone wounds.
[d]Unless primary immunization was "fluid" rather than absorbed vaccine.

References
1. Abrutyn E: Tetanus. In general reference 1, p 577.
2. Brand DA, et al: Adequacy of Antitetanus Prophylaxis in Six Hospital Emergency Rooms. *N Engl J Med* 309:636, 1983.
3. Cate TR: *Clostridium tetani* (Tetanus). In Mandell GL, et al (eds): *Principles and Practice of Infectious Diseases* (3rd ed). New York: Churchill Livingstone, 1993, p 1842.
4. Centers for Disease Control: Diphtheria, Tetanus, and Pertussis: Guidelines for Vaccine Prophylaxis and Other Preventive Measures. *Ann Intern Med* 103:896, 1985.
5. Furste W: Four Keys to 100 Percent Success in Tetanus Prophylaxis. *Am J Surg* 128:616, 1974.

3-D. Selected Venereal Diseases: Current Treatment Recommendations

Gonorrhea

Diagnosis	Recommended treatment
Gonococcal infection in men and women	Ceftriaxone, 250 mg IM OR Ciprofloxacin,[a] 500 mg once PO OR Ofloxacin,[a] 400 mg once PO OR Cefixime,[b] 400 mg once PO OR Spectinomycin,[c] 2 gm IM once PLUS Tetracycline,[a] 500 mg PO qid for 7 days, or doxycycline[a] 100 mg PO bid for 7 days

	OR
	For patients in whom tetracyclines are contraindicated or not tolerated, the single dose regimen may be followed by erythromycin base or stearate, 500 mg PO qid for 7 days, or erythromycin ethylsuccinate 800 mg PO qid for 7 days
Acute salpingitis (pelvic inflammatory disease)	
Outpatients	Ampicillin, 3.5 gm PO; or amoxicillin, 3.0 gm PO; or procaine penicillin, 4.8 million units IM in two divided doses, each with probenecid, 1 gm PO, followed by doxycycline,[a] 100 mg PO bid for 10–14 days.
	OR
	Ceftriaxone, 250 mg IM and doxycycline,[a] 100 mg PO bid for 10–14 days.
	Metronidazole, 500 mg PO qid for 10–14 days may be added in severe cases.
Hospitalized patients (at least 4 days of IV and 14 days of total therapy)	Doxycycline,[a] 100 mg IV q12h; cefoxitin, 2 gm IV q6h; followed by doxycycline,[a] 100 mg PO bid
	OR
	Clindamycin, 900 mg IV q8h; gentamicin, 2 mg/kg IV once, followed by 1.5 mg/kg IV q8h;[c] followed by clindamycin, 450 mg PO qid or doxycycline,[a] 100 mg PO bid

3-D. Selected Venereal Diseases: Current Treatment Recommendations (continued)

Gonorrhea

Diagnosis	Recommended treatment
Disseminated gonococcal infection (arthritis-dermatitis syndrome)	Ceftriaxone, 1 gm IV or IM q24h OR Cefotaxime, 1 gm IV q8h OR Ceftizoxime, 1 gm IV q8h In β-lactam allergic patients, spectinomycin, 2 gm IM q12h Reliable patients may be discharged 24 hours after symptoms resolve to complete 10 days therapy with: Cefuroxime axetil, 500 mg PO bid OR Ampicillin/clavulinic acid, 500 mg PO tid OR Cefixime[b], 400 mg PO qd Consider concomitant chlamydia therapy

Nongonococcal urethritis	Doxycycline,[a] 100 gm PO bid for 7 days
	OR
	Tetracycline,[a] 500 mg PO qid for 7 days
	OR
	Erythromycin, 500 mg PO qid for 7–21 days
	OR
	Azithromycin,[a] 1 gm PO single dose

3-D. Selected Venereal Diseases: Current Treatment Recommendations (continued)

Syphilis

Diagnosis/stage	Recommended treatment[e]	
	Non–penicillin-allergic	Penicillin-allergic
Primary, secondary, or early latent	Penicillin G benzathine, 2.4 million units IM (half in each hip) as single dose OR Penicillin G procaine, 600,000 units IM qd for 8 days	Erythromycin or tetracycline,[a] 500 mg PO qid, or doxycycline,[a] 100 mg PO bid for 14 days
Late latent, latent of undetermined duration, cardiovascular, benign tertiary	Penicillin G benzathine, 2.4 million units IM once a week for 3 weeks	Erythromycin or tetracycline,[a] 500 mg PO qid for 30 days, or doxycycline,[a] 100 mg PO bid for 30 days

| Neurosyphilis | Aqueous crystalline penicillin G, 2.4 million units IV q4h for 10 days; or penicillin G procaine, 2.4 million units IM qd, and probenecid, 500 mg PO qid, both for 10 days PLUS Penicillin G benzathine, 2.4 million units IM once a week for 3 weeks | Erythromycin or tetracycline[a] 500 mg PO qid for 30 days, or doxycycline,[a] 100 mg PO bid for 30 days |
| In pregnancy | Same as for nonpregnant, according to stage | Skin test for penicillin allergy; desensitize if necessary |

[a]Contraindicated in pregnancy.
[b]Efficacy in pregnancy not established.
[c]Ineffective in pharyngeal infection.
[d]Dose modification may be required in renal insufficiency.
[e]In HIV-positive patients, modified treatment regimens may be indicated.

References
1. Drugs for sexually transmitted diseases. *Med Lett Drugs Ther* 33:119, 1991.
2. Sanford JP: *Guide to Antimicrobial Therapy.* Dallas: Antimicrobial Therapy, Inc., 1993, p 14.
3. Tramont ED: *Treponema Pallidum* (Syphilis). In Mandell GL, et al. (eds): *Principles and Practice of Infectious Diseases* (3rd ed). New York: Churchill Livingstone, 1990, p 1794.

3-E. Common Drugs Requiring Dosage Adjustment in Renal Failure

Antibiotics
Acyclovir
Amantadine
Aminoglycosides (e.g., tobramycin)
Amphotericin
Ampicillin
Aztreonam
Cephalosporins (except cefoperazone, ceftriaxone)
Chloroquine
Ciprofloxacin
Clarithromycin
Cycloserine
Doxycycline
Ethambutol
Fluconazole
5-Fluorocytosine
Ganciclovir
Imipenem
Isoniazid (especially slow acetylators)
Metronidazole
Nalidixic acid
Nitrofurantoin
Norfloxacin
Ofloxacin
Penicillins (except cloxacillin, dicloxacillin, nafcillin, oxacillin)
Pentamidine
Pyrazinamide
Ribavirin
Sulfamethoxazole-trimethoprim
Sulfisoxazole

Tetracylines (except minocycline)
Trimethoprim
Vancomycin
Zidovudine

Analgesics
Acetaminophen
Aspirin
Butorphanol
Codeine
Fentanyl
Meperidine
Methadone
Morphine
Pentazocine
Phenazopyridine (Pyridium)
Propoxyphene (Darvon)

Sedatives and Psychiatric Drugs
Buspirone
Chlordiazepoxide (Librium)
Chloral hydrate
Ethchlorvynol
Glutethimide (Doriden)
Lithium carbonate
Lorazepam
Meprobamate
Methaqualone
Midazolam
Phenobarbital

Cardiovascular Drugs
Acebutolol
Acetazolamide
Amiloride
Atenolol
Betaxolol
Bretylium
Captopril
Chlorthalidone
Clonidine
Digitoxin (for creatinine clearance < 10 ml/min)
Digoxin
Disopyramide (Norpace)
Enalapril
Ethacrynic acid
Flecainide

Guanethidine
Hydralazine
Lisinopril
Methyldopa
Mexiletine
Moricizine
Nadolol
Nitroprusside
Procainamide
Propafenone
Quinapril
Ramipril
Reserpine
Sotalol
Spironolactone
Thiazides
Tocainide
Triamterene
Verapamil

Antineoplastic and Immunosuppressive Drugs
Azathioprine
Bleomycin
Cisplatin
Cyclophosphamide
Daunorubicin
Doxorubicin
Etoposide
Fludarabine
Hydroxyurea
Melphalan
Methotrexate
Mitomycin C
Nitrosourea
Plicamycin
Streptozotocin

Arthritic Drugs
Acetaminophen
Allopurinol
Aspirin
Colchicine
Diflunisal
Gold
Ketorolac

Penicillamine
Phenylbutazone
Probenecid
Sulfinpyrazone
Sulindac

Anticonvulsants
Carbamazepine (Tegretol)
Ethosuximide
Phenobarbital
Primidone
Trimethadione
Valproic acid

Miscellaneous Agents
Baclofen
Cimetidine
Clofibrate
Diphenhydramine (Benadryl)
Famotidine
Gallamine (Flaxedil)
Gemfibrozil
Hypoglycemic agents
   Acetohexamide (Dymelor)
   Chlorpropamide (Diabinese)
   Insulin
   Tolbutamide (Orinase)
Magnesium antacids
Metoclopramide
Neostigmine
Nicotinic acid
Nizatidine
Pancuronium
Propylthiouracil
Ranitidine
Terbutaline (especially parenteral)

References
1. Miller SB: Dosage Adjustments of Drugs in Renal Failure. In general reference 2, p 529.
2. Bennett WM, et al: Drug Prescribing in Renal Failure: Philadelphia: American College of Physicians, 1991.
3. Schrier RW, Gambertoglio JG (eds): *Handbook of Drug Therapy in Liver and Kidney Disease.* Boston: Little, Brown, 1991.

3-F. Guidelines for Intravenous Aminophylline Therapy*

Loading dose

	Dose (mg/kg)[a]
No known theophylline ingestion in past 24–48 hr	5–6 mg/kg over 15–30 min[b]
Theophylline ingested within past 48 hr	0–4 mg/kg over 15–30 min[c]
Poor clinical response to initial loading dose and no clinical signs of toxicity, or theophylline blood level < 15 μg/ml	Additional 1–3 mg/kg over 15–30 min

[a]Based on ideal body weight.
[b]To raise serum level by 10 μg/ml.
[c]Therapy is guided by theophylline blood level, if available.

Maintenance dose (continuous infusion)*

	Dose (mg/kg/hr)[a,b]
Children > 9 yr old and adult smokers < 55 yr old	0.50–0.90
Adult nonsmokers	0.40–0.60
Severe airway obstruction	0.40
Mild-to-moderate heart failure	≤ 0.40
Severe heart failure	≤0.20
Pneumonia	0.20–0.40
Liver dysfunction with serum bilirubin < 1.5 mg/dl and serum albumin > 2.9 gm/dl	≤ 0.45
Liver dysfunction with serum bilirubin > 1.5 mg/dl and/or serum albumin < 2.9 gm/dl	≤ 0.20

[a]Adolescents and/or smokers generally metabolize theophylline more rapidly and often receive higher doses.
[b]Patients taking propranolol, isoniazid, calcium channel blockers, mexiletine, caffeine, erythromycin, cimetidine, troleandomycin (Tao), thiabendazole, mebendazole, ciprofloxacin, allopurinol, oral contraceptives, norfloxacin, or ofloxacin metabolize theophylline more slowly and may require a reduction in dosage. Patients taking phenytoin, phenobarbital, carbamazepine, furosemide, or rifampin may require an increase in dosage.

References

1. Hendeles L, Weinberger M: Poisoning Patients with Intravenous Theophylline (editorial). *Am J Hosp Pharm* 37:49, 1980.
2. Powell JR, et al: Theophylline Disposition in Acutely Ill Hospitalized Patients. *Am Rev Respir Dis* 118:229, 1978.
3. Hendeles L, Weinberger M, Bighley L: Disposition of Theophylline after a Single Intravenous Infusion of Aminophylline. *Am Rev Respir Dis* 118:97, 1978.

*Serum theophylline determinations after 12–36 hr of continuous aminophylline infusion are useful.

3-G. Dopamine and Dobutamine Dosage Charts

Dopamine (Intropin) 800 mg/500 ml = 1.6 mg/ml

Weight		Dosage (μg/kg/min)*							
lb	kg	1.0	2.5	5.0	7.5	10.0	12.5	15.0	20.0
88	40	2	4	7	11	15	19	22	30
99	45	2	4	8	12	17	20	25	34
110	50	2	5	9	14	19	23	28	38
121	55	2	5	10	15	22	25	31	42
132	60	3	6	11	17	23	28	34	46
143	65	3	6	12	18	25	30	36	49
154	70	4	7	13	20	26	33	39	52
165	75	4	7	14	21	28	35	42	57
176	80	4	8	15	22	30	38	45	60
187	85	4	8	16	23	32	40	48	64
198	90	4	9	17	25	34	42	51	68
209	95	5	9	18	26	36	45	53	72
220	100	5	10	19	27	38	47	57	76

*Flow rate in drops/min; based on a microdrip: 60 drops/min = 1 ml.
Source: Freitag JJ, Miller LW (eds): *Manual of Medical Therapeutics* (23rd ed). Boston: Little, Brown, 1980, app IV, p 455.

Dobutamine (Dobutrex) 500 mg (2 vials)/500 ml = 1.0 mg/ml

Weight		Dosage (µg/kg/min)*							
lb	kg	1.0	2.5	5.0	7.5	10.0	12.5	15.0	20.0
88	40	2	5	11	16	22	29	36	45
99	45	3	7	14	20	27	34	41	54
110	50	3	8	15	23	30	38	45	60
121	55	3	8	17	25	33	41	50	66
132	60	4	9	18	27	36	45	54	72
143	65	4	10	20	29	39	49	59	78
154	70	4	11	21	32	42	53	63	84
165	75	5	11	23	34	45	56	68	90
176	80	5	12	24	36	48	60	72	96
187	85	5	13	26	38	51	64	77	102
198	90	5	14	27	41	54	68	81	108
209	95	6	14	29	43	57	71	86	114
220	100	6	15	30	45	60	75	90	120

*Flow rate in drops/min; based on a microdrip: 60 drops = 1 ml.
Source: Freitag J, Miller LW (eds): *Manual of Medical Therapeutics* (23rd ed). Boston: Little, Brown, 1980, app V, p 456.

3-H. Glucocorticoid Preparations

USP name	Trade name	Tablet size (mg)	Relative antiinflammatory potency	Relative mineralocorticoid potency	Approximate equivalent dose (mg)	Biologic half-life (hr)[a]
Short-acting						
Hydrocortisone (cortisol)	Hydrocortone, Solu-Cortef[b]	5, 10, 20	1.0	1.0	20.0	8–12
Cortisone		5, 10, 20	0.8	0.8	25.0	8–12
Intermediate-acting						
Prednisone	Deltasone	1, 2.5, 5, 10, 20, 50	4.0	0.8	5.0	12–36
Prednisolone	Hydeltrasol[b]	5	4.0	0.8	5.0	12–36
Methylprednisolone	Medrol, Solu-Medrol[b]	2, 4, 8, 16, 24, 32	5.0	0.5	4.0	12–36

Triamcinolone	Aristocort, Aristospan[b]		5.0	0	4.0	12–36
Long-acting						
Dexamethasone	Decadron, Dalalone[b]	0.25, 0.5, 0.75, 1.5, 4	25	0	0.75	36–72
Betamethasone	Celestone	0.6	25	0	0.60	36–72

[a] Apply to only oral and intravenous routes of administration.
[b] Parenteral form.
Source: Modified from Kahl LE: Arthritis and Rheumatologic Diseases. In general reference 2, p 452.

References

1. Haynes RC: Adrenocorticotropic Hormone, Adrenocortical Steroids and Their Synthetic Analogs; Inhibitors of the Synthesis and Actions of Adrenocortical Hormones. In Gilman AG, et al (eds). *The Pharmacological Basis of Therapeutics* (8th ed). New York: Pergamon, 1990, p 1431.

2. Axelrod L: Glucocorticoid Therapy. *Medicine* 55:39, 1976.

3-I. Hypoglycemic Agents

Characteristics of commonly used insulin preparations*

Classification	Insulin preparation	Action		
		Onset	Peak	Duration (hr)
Rapid-acting	Regular	IV: immediate	15–30 min	2
		IM: 5–30 min	30–60 min	2–4
		SC: 15–60 min	2–6 hr	4–12
	Semilente	SC: 30–60 min	3–10 hr	8–18
Intermediate-acting	NPH	SC: 1.5–4 hr	6–16 hr	12–24
	Lente	SC: 1–4 hr	6–16 hr	12–28
Slow-acting	Protamine zinc insulin (PZI)	SC: 3–8 hr	14–26 hr	24–40
	Ultralente	SC: 3–8 hr	8–28 hr	24–40
Mixed insulin	Novolin 70/30	30 min	2–12 hr	24

*Activity may be prolonged in renal failure.
Source: Modified from Orland MJ: Diabetes Mellitus. In general reference 2, p 382.

Oral hypoglycemic agents (sulfonylureas)*

Type	Available form (mg)	Total daily dose (mg)	Duration of action (hr)	Dose given
Tolbutamide (Orinase)	250, 500	500–3000	6–12	bid–tid
Chlorpropamide (Diabinese)	100, 250	100–500	up to 90	qd–bid
Tolazamide (Tolinase)	100, 250, 500	100–1000	12–24	qd–bid
Glipizide (Glucotrol)	5, 10	5–40	12–24	qd–bid
Glyburide (DiaBeta, Micronase)	1.25, 2.5, 5	2.5–20	24–60	qd–bid

*Activity is prolonged in both hepatic and renal failure.
Source: Modified from Orland MJ: Diabetes Mellitus. In general reference 2, p. 375.

Factors Causing Hyperglycemia in Diabetics

Weight gain or increased carbohydrate ingestion
Intravenous carbohydrate infusion (e.g., hyperalimentation)
Pubertal growth
Pregnancy
Nonuse or incorrect use of insulin
Infection or inflammation
Ketoacidosis
Emotional stress
Other acute stress (e.g., myocardial infarction, pancreatitis,
    surgery)
Endocrinopathies
  Hyperthyroidism
  Pheochromocytoma
  Hyperadrenocorticism
  Profound hyperlipidemia
  Primary hyperparathyroidism
  Acromegaly
Decreased activity or exercise
Pancreatic disease or resection
Drug-induced pancreatic islet cell destruction (e.g., strepto-
    zocin, pentamidine isethionate)
Hypokalemia
Hypomagnesemia
Drugs
  Nicotinic acid
  Diazoxide
  Sympathomimetics
  Glucocorticoids
  Phenytoin
  Thyroid hormone preparations
  Diuretics
  Oral contraceptives
Change in oral hypoglycemic therapy
Insulin or insulin-receptor antibodies
Insulin-resistant states

Factors Causing Hypoglycemia in Diabetics

Weight reduction or decreased carbohydrate ingestion
Decreased intravenous carbohydrate infusion
Increased activity
Overdose of insulin and/or sulfonylurea therapy
Drug interactions with sulfonylurea therapy
  Warfarin
  Salicylates
  Chloramphenicol

Clofibrate
Sulfonamides
Methyldopa
Miconazole
Phenylbutazone
Probenecid
Monoamine oxidase inhibitors
Renal insufficiency
Alcohol ingestion
Hypothyroidism
Hypoadrenocorticism
Decreased dosage or discontinuation of drugs (e.g., gluco-
    corticoids, diuretics, thyroid hormone preparations)
Intercurrent processes causing hypoglycemia (e.g., insulin-
    oma; see 4-J)

References
1. Orland MJ: Diabetes Mellitus. In general reference 2, p
   375.
2. Foster DW, Rubenstein AH: Hypoglycemia. In general
   reference 1, p 1759.

3-J. Selected Intravenous Vasoactive Drugs

Drug	Common preparations	Dosage	Comments
Dopamine (Intropin)	1 amp = 200–800 mg; add 800 mg to 250–500 ml 5% D/W or NS	Initial dose: 1–4 µg/kg/min; titrate to effect	Doses > 12–14 µg/kg/min cause primarily alpha-adrenergic effects (e.g., vasoconstriction); doses < 10 µg/kg/min cause mainly beta-adrenergic effects (e.g., increased stroke volume) and increased renal blood flow
Dobutamine (Dobutrex)	1 amp = 250 mg; add 500 mg to 250–500 ml 5% D/W or NS	Initial dose: 1–4 µg/kg/min; titrate to effect	Doses > 20 µg/kg/min may be associated with arrhythmias
Isoproterenol (Isuprel)	1 amp = 1 mg; add 1–2 mg to 500 ml 5% D/W or NS	Initial dose: 1 µg/min; titrate to effect	Doses > 10 µg/min may be associated with arrhythmias
Norepinephrine (Levophed)	1 amp = 4 mg; add 4–8 mg to 500 ml 5% DW only	Initial dose: 2–15 µg/min; titrate to effect	Mainly alpha-adrenergic effects (i.e., vasoconstriction) in most vascular beds

Amrinone (Inocor)	1 amp = 100 mg; dilute to 1–3 mg/ml concentration in saline solution. Do not use dextrose	Initial dose: 0.75 mg/kg over 2–3 min and then infuse continuously 5–10 μg/kg/min	Side effects: thrombocytopenia, gastrointestinal upset, fever, myalgia, hepatic dysfunction, ventricular irritability, and hypotension
Sodium nitroprusside (Nipride)	1 amp = 50 mg; add 50–100 mg to 250 ml 5% D/W only	Initial dose: 0.3–5 μg/kg/min; titrate to effect only or maximum of 10 μg/kg/min; average effective dose is 3 μg/kg/min	Infusion apparatus must be shielded from light; infusion pump is required; total dose > 3 mg/kg may be associated with toxicity, especially when renal insufficiency is present
Milrinone (Primacor)	50 mg in 200 ml 5% D/W or NS	Initial dose: 50 μg/kg slow IVP over 10 min and then infuse continuously 0.375–0.750 μg/kg/min; titrate to effect	Side effects: hypotension, ventricular arrhythmias, headaches
Nitroglycerin	Usually 1 amp = 50 mg; add 50 mg to 250 ml 5% D/W or NS; follow supplier's recommendations	Initial dose: 3–10 μg/min. Increase by 5–10 μg/min every 3–5 min until response seen. Usual maximum dose: 300 μg/min	Use glass bottles and nonabsorbing tubing. Treat hypotension with volume and cessation of infusion

3-J. Selected Intravenous Vasoactive Drugs (continued)

Drug	Common preparations	Dosage	Comments
Bretylium (Bretylol)	1 amp = 500 mg; add 2 gm to 500 ml 5% D/W or NS	For ventricular tachycardia, 5–10 mg/kg (undiluted) IVP over 10 min then infuse continuously 1–4 mg/min	Hypotension and/or arrhythmias may be provoked
Procainamide	10 ml vial = 1000 mg; 2 ml vial = 1000 mg; add 2 gm to 500 ml 5% D/W or NS	Loading dose: < 15 mg/kg IVPB at < 50 mg/min; then infuse continuously 1–5 mg/min	Hypotension is main toxicity
Lidocaine	1 amp = 50 or 100 mg; premix 2 g in 500 ml 5% D/W	Initial dose: 50–100 mg IVP; may repeat after 5 min then infuse continuously 1–4 mg/min	No more than 200–300 mg of lidocaine should be administered in a 1 hr period

NS = normal saline, IVP = IV push; IVPB = IV piggyback.

References

1. Kelly DP, Fry ETA: Heart failure. In general reference 2, p 105.
2. Weil MH, Planta MV, Rackow EC: Acute Circulatory Failure (Shock). In general reference 7, p 569.
3. *Physicians' Desk Reference*. Montvale, NJ: Medical Economics Data, 1993.

3-K. Drug and Disease Interactions with Warfarin (Coumadin)

Increased Prothrombin Time

Acetaminophen
Age
Alcohol*
Allopurinol
Amiodarone
Anabolic steroids
Antibiotics
Bromelains
Cancer
Chloral hydrate*
Chlorpropamide
Cholestyramine*
Chymotrypsin
Cimetidine
Ciprofloxacin
Clofibrate
Collagen vascular disease
Congestive heart failure
Dextran
Dextrothyroxine
Diarrhea
Diazoxide
Diflunisal
Disulfiram
Diuretics*
Ethacrynic acid
Fenoprofen
Fever
Fluconazole
Gemfibrozil
Glucagon
Heparin
Hepatic disease

Hepatotoxic drugs
Hyperthyroidism
Hypoglycemic agents
Ibuprofen
Indomethacin
Influenza vaccine
Inhalation anesthetics
Itraconazole
Ketoconazole
Malnutrition
Mefenamic acid
Methyldopa
Methylphenidate
Metronidazole
Miconazole
Monoamine oxidase inhibitors
Nalidixic acid
Naproxen
Narcotics
Norfloxacin
Oxyphenbutazone
Pentoxifylline
Phenylbutazone
Phenytoin
Propoxyphene
Propylthiouracil
Pyrazolones
Quinidine
Quinine
Ranitidine
Salicylates (> 1 gm daily)
Sulfinpyrazone
Sulfonamides
Sulindac
Tamoxifen
Thyroid preparations
Tolbutamide
Tricyclic antidepressants
Trimethoprim-sulfamethoxazole
Vitamin K malabsorption or deficiency

Decreased Prothrombin Time
Alcohol*
Aluminum hydroxide
Antihistamines
Barbiturates
Carbamazepine

Chloral hydrate*
Chlordiazepoxide
Cholestyramine*
Diuretics*
Edema
Estrogens
Ethchlorvynol
Glucocorticoids
Glutethimide
Griseofulvin
Haloperidol
Hereditary resistance
Insecticides
Meprobamate
Myxedema
Nafcillin
Nephrotic syndrome
Oral contraceptives
Paraldehyde
Pregnancy (mother only)
Prolonged hot weather
Primidone
Ranitidine
Rifampin
Sucralfate
Trazodone
Vitamin C
Vitamin K

References
1. *Physicians' Desk Reference.* Montvale, NJ: Medical Economics Data, 1993, p 963.
2. Lentz SR: Disorders of Hemostasis. In general reference 2, p 338.
3. Majerus PW, et al: Anticoagulant, Thrombolytic, and Anti-Platelet Drugs. In Gilman AG, et al (eds). *The Pharmacological Basis of Therapeutics* (8th ed). New York: Pergamon, 1990, p 1311.

*Can cause increased or decreased prothrombin time.

3-L. Partial List of Drugs Used During Pregnancy at Barnes Hospital

Type of medication	Safe to use in pregnancy[a]	Limited information, relatively safe[b]	Risks associated with use[c]	Avoid in pregnancy[d]
Analgesics	Acetaminophen	Hydromorphone[e] Codeine[e] Meperidine[e] Oxycodone with aspirin[e] Morphine[e]	Salicylates Ibuprofen Indomethacin	

Antibiotics	Ampicillin Erythromycin Penicillin Carbenicillin	Amikacin Amphotericin B Nitrofurantoin Ampicillin with sulbactam Amoxicillin with clavulanic acid Miconazole Aztreonam Ticarcillin Oxacillin Methicillin Cephalosporins Clindamycin Gentamicin Tobramycin	Chloramphenicol Metronidazole Isoniazid Streptomycin Sulfonamides Rifampin Trimethoprim Kanamycin	Chloroquine Ciprofloxacin Norfloxacin Tetracyclines
Anticoagulants		Dipyridamole Heparin		Warfarin
Antiemetics		Meclizine Trimethobenzamide Metoclopramide	Thiethylperazine Prochlorperazine	

3-L. Partial List of Drugs Used During Pregnancy at Barnes Hospital (continued)

Type of medication	Safe to use in pregnancy[a]	Limited information, relatively safe[b]	Risks associated with use[c]	Avoid in pregnancy[d]
Antiepileptics		Ethosuximide	Clonazepam Phenytoin Valproic acid Primidone Phenobarbital	
Antihistamines	Tripelennamine		Brompheniramine Terfenadine Astemizole Diphenhydramine	Hydroxyzine
Antihypertensives		Hydralazine Methyldopa Clonidine Metoprolol Prazosin	Atenolol Nitroprusside Diazoxide Labetalol Timolol Propranolol Nadolol	Captopril Reserpine Enalapril Lisinopril

Asthma preparations		Beclomethasone Aminophylline Cromolyn sodium Terbutaline Ipratropium bromide	Albuterol Isoproterenol Metaproterenol
Cardiac drugs	Digoxin	Procainamide Atropine Quinidine Lidocaine Verapamil Disopyramide	Diltiazem Nifedipine
Cough preparations		Terpin hydrate Guaifenesin	
Diuretics†	Furosemide	Bumetanide Ethacrynic acid Acetazolamide Hydrochloro- thiazide	

3-L. Partial List of Drugs Used During Pregnancy at Barnes Hospital (continued)

Type of medication	Safe to use in pregnancy[a]	Limited information, relatively safe[b]	Risks associated with use[c]	Avoid in pregnancy[d]
Hypoglycemics[g]	Insulin			Chlorpropamide Tolbutamide Glyburide
Laxatives	Milk of magnesia Psyllium	Docusate		
Sedatives				Barbiturates Benzodiazepines
Thyroid preparations	Thyroxine		Methimazole Propylthiouracil Iodide	
Other drugs	Ferrous sulfate Kaopectate Probenecid Antacids	Allopurinol Clofibrate H₂ antagonists Vaccines (influenza, polio, rabies, tetanus)	Glucocorticoids Amphetamines EDTA General anesthesia drugs Haloperidol Penicillamine	Antineoplastic agents Bromocriptine Lithium Disulfiram Estrogens, diethylstil-bestrol

Phenothiazines	Isotretinoin
	Quinine
	Tricyclic antidepressants
	Vaccines (rubella, mumps, measles, smallpox)
	Misoprostol

aAlthough no drug can be used with certainty that there will be no adverse effects, drugs listed in this column are used at Barnes Hospital.
bMany drugs in this column are new and data are limited, but no consistent adverse effect has been attributed to their use.
cThese drugs have some associated risk when used in pregnancy. The potential benefit must be weighed against possible adverse effects.
dThese drugs have been well documented to produce adverse fetal effects. They should not be used in pregnancy.
ePossible neonatal addiction and withdrawal may occur after long-term use. Neonatal depression may occur with intrapartum use.
fDiuretics can deplete maternal intravascular volume and, in rare instances, can be associated with neonatal thrombocytopenia. Diuretics are not indicated in pregnancy-induced hypertension as first-line agents.
gThere is no place for oral hypoglycemic agents in the treatment of diabetes in pregnancy. Oral hypoglycemic agents have been associated with prolonged hypoglycemia in newborn infants. Insulin and dietary control are indicated to bring blood sugar under rigid control.
Source: From Pitman, AM. In Woodley M, Whelan A (eds): *Manual of Medical Therepeutics* (27th ed). Boston: Little, Brown, 1992, pp 539–541.

4 ENDOCRINE/ METABOLIC SYSTEM

4-A. Amenorrhea

Hypothalamic and Pituitary Causes
Hypothalamic-pituitary dysfunction with hyperprolactinemia
(see 4-C)
  Drugs (e.g., phenothiazines)
  Prolactinomas
  Primary hypothyroidism
Hypothalamic-pituitary dysfunction due to extrinsic factors
  Nutritional
    Obesity
    Weight loss (including anorexia nervosa)
  Strenuous exercise
  Stress
  Pseudocyesis
  Post-pill amenorrhea
  Chronic debilitating diseases (e.g., poorly-controlled dia-
      betes mellitus, uremia, rheumatoid arthritis)
  Cushing's syndrome
  Hypothyroidism
  Late-onset congenital adrenal hyperplasia
  Lactation
  Pregnancy
  Anovulation

Hypothalamic-pituitary dysfunction due to intrinsic factors
    Amenorrhea and anosmia
    Empty-sella syndrome
    Hypopituitarism/hypothalamic disease (see 4-Q)

Ovarian Causes

With decreased ovarian steroid production
    Congenital
        Gonadal agenesis
        Resistant ovary syndrome (Savage syndrome)
        Gonadal dysgenesis (including Turner's syndrome)
        Sex chromosome mosaicism
        XY gonadal dysgenesis
        17α-Hydroxylase deficiency
        True hermaphroditism
    Acquired: premature primary ovarian failure
        Autoimmune
        Chemotherapy
        Radiation
        Surgical castration
        Postinfection (e.g., mumps)
        Severe pelvic inflammatory disease
    Menopause
With increased ovarian steroid production
    Feminizing ovarian tumors
    Masculinizing ovarian tumors
    Polycystic ovary syndrome

Uterine and Outflow Tract Abnormalities

Hysterectomy
Müllerian agenesis
Müllerian anomalies
    Labial agglutination or fusion
    Imperforate hymen
    Absence or anomalies of vagina, cervix, or uterus
Trauma
    Cervical stenosis
    Vaginal stenosis
    Sclerosis of uterine cavity (Asherman's syndrome)
        Following postabortal or postpartum infection or
            trauma
        Following myomectomy or cesarean section
        Severe endometritis (including tuberculous endometritis)
Male pseudohermaphroditism
    Testicular feminization
    5α-Reductase deficiency

Female pseudohermaphroditism
  Congenital adrenal hyperplasia
  Exposure to maternal androgens in utero

References

1. Speroff L, Glass RH, Kase NG: *Clinical Gynecologic Endocrinology and Infertility.* (4th ed). Baltimore: Williams & Wilkins, 1989, p 80–204.
2. Reindollar RH, et al: Adult-Onset Amenorrhea: A Study of 262 Patients. *Am J Obstet Gynecol* 155:531, 1986.

4-B. Gynecomastia

Pseudogynecomastia
  Obesity
  Benign or malignant breast tumor
Physiologic
  Newborn
  Adolescence
  Normal physical finding
  Old age
Familial gynecomastia
Persistent pubertal macromastia
Deficient testosterone production or action
  End organ insensitivity to androgens
    Testicular feminization
    Reifenstein's syndrome
  Primary hypogonadism
    Klinefelter's syndrome
    Congenital anorchia
    XX males
    Orchitis
      Viral
      Neisseria gonorrhoeae
      Granulomatous (especially leprosy)
    Irradiation
    Trauma
    Castration
    Associated with neurologic disease
      Myotonia atrophica
      Spinal cord disease
    Defects in testosterone synthesis
    Uremia

Secondary or tertiary hypogonadism (rarely)
    Kallmann's syndrome
    Hypopituitarism/hypothalamic disease (see 4-Q)
Neoplasms
    Producing estrogens or estrogen precursors
        Feminizing adrenal tumors
        Testicular tumors
    Secreting human chorionic gonadotropin (HCG)
        Germinal cell tumors of the testicle
        Nontesticular tumors
            Gynecomastia reported with elevated HCG
                Undifferentiated mediastinal carcinoma
                Adenocarcinoma of the stomach
                Hepatoma, hepatoblastoma
                Carcinoma of the pancreas
                Carcinoma of the lung
            Detectable HCG reported without gynecomastia (so far)
                Lymphoma
                Melanoma
                Esophagus
                Biliary tract
                Small intestine
                Liver sarcoma
                Colon/rectal
                Leukemia
                Multiple myeloma
                Sarcomas
                Breast
                Insulinoma
                Pheochromocytoma
                Renal cell carcinoma
                Medullary carcinoma of the thyroid
    Secreting prolactin
        Pituitary prolactinomas
    Secreting gonadotropins
        Gonadotropin-secreting pituitary adenomas
Increased estrogen production
    True hermaphroditism
        Inherited increased peripheral aromatase activity
    Increased availability of estrogen precursors
        Liver disease (especially cirrhosis)
        Thyrotoxicosis
        Congenital adrenal hyperplasia
            11-Hydroxylase deficiency
            21-Hydroxylase deficiency
Systemic diseases (especially recovery from chronic disease)
    Refeeding gynecomastia (following starvation)

Poorly controlled diabetes mellitus
Pulmonary tuberculosis
Drugs
  Amiodarone
  Amphetamines
  Androgens
  Calcium channel blockers
  Captopril
  Cimetidine
  Clomiphene
  Cytotoxic agents
    Busulfan
    Cisplatin
    Nitrosoureas
    Vincristine
    Combination chemotherapy
  Diazepam
  Diethylpropion
  Digitalis
  Estrogens
  Ethionamide
  Etomidate
  Flutamide
  Gonadotropins
  Heroin
  Isoniazid
  Ketoconazole
  Marijuana
  Methyldopa
  Metronidazole
  Omeprazole
  Penicillamine
  Phenothiazines
  Phenytoin
  Reserpine
  Spironolactone
  Tricyclic antidepressants
Idiopathic gynecomastia

References
1. Braunstein GD: Gynecomastia. *N Engl J Med* 328:490, 1993.
2. Carlson HE: Gynecomastia: Pathogenesis and Therapy. *The Endocrinologist* 1:337, 1991.

4-C. Galactorrhea

Without hyperprolactinemia
  Pseudogalactorrhea
    Intramammary lesions
      Benign
        Fibrocystic disease
        Intraductal papilloma
      Malignant neoplasm
  Idiopathic galactorrhea with menses
  Post–oral contraceptive galactorrhea
With hyperprolactinemia
  Drugs
    Neuroleptics
      Phenothiazines
      Thioxanthenes
      Butyrophenones
      Diphenylbutylpiperidines
      Dihydroindolones
    Cocaine
    Reserpine
    Alpha-methyldopa
    Opiates
    Substituted benzamides
      Sulpiride
      Metoclopramide
      Celebropride
      Brompride
    Antidepressants
      Tricyclic antidepressants
      Dibenzoxazepine antidepressants
      Amoxapine
    Estrogens
    Cimetidine
    Verapamil
    Benzodiazepines
    Androgens
    Isoniazid
    Meprobamate
    Amphetamines
  Diseases affecting the hypothalamus and/or pituitary
          stalk
    Central nervous system sarcoidosis
    Craniopharyngiomas
    Pinealomas
    Aneurysms
    Hypothalamic tumors, primary or metastatic

Pituitary stalk section (including tumors compressing
     the stalk)
Encephalitis/postencephalitis
Basilar meningitis
Pseudotumor cerebri
Post-pneumoencephalogram
Schüller-Christian disease
Hydrocephalus
Neuraxis irradiation
Other destructive lesions of the hypothalamus (see
     4-Q)
Tumors secreting prolactin or placental lactogen
   Prolactinomas
   Acromegaly
   Bronchogenic carcinoma
   Hypernephroma
   Uterine leiomyomas
   Chorionepithelioma
   Hydatidiform mole
Cirrhosis
Empty-sella syndrome
Primary hypothyroidism
Pregnancy
Chronic renal failure
Refeeding after starvation
Addison's disease
Neural stimulation
Disorders of the chest wall and thorax
   Thoracotomy
   Mastectomy/mammoplasty
   Thoracoplasty
   Burns
   Herpes zoster
   Bronchogenic tumors
   Bronchiectasis/chronic bronchitis
   Neoplasms of the chest wall
   Chest wall injury
Nipple stimulation
   Chronic inflammatory disease
   Mechanical stimulation of the nipples
Spinal cord
   Tabes dorsalis
   Syringomyelia
   Cervical spinal cord lesions
Psychogenic
   Pseudocyesis
   Stresses
   Posttrauma

Major surgery and anesthesia, especially including
oophorectomy
Idiopathic hyperprolactinemia

References

1. Kleinberg DL, Noel GC, Frantz AG: Galactorrhea: A
   Study of 235 Cases, Including 48 with Pituitary Tumors.
   N Engl J Med 296:589, 1977.
2. Speroff S, Glass RH, Kase NG: *Clinical Gynecologic En-
   docrinology and Infertility* (4th ed). Baltimore: Williams &
   Wilkins, 1989, pp 291–294.

4-D. Hypothermia

Accidental hypothermia
   Environmental exposure (especially in neonates, prema-
      ture or low-birth-weight babies, elderly, or persons who
      are unconscious, immobilized, drugged, or exhausted)
   Cold-water immersion
Endocrine disorders
   Hypothyroidism
   Hypoglycemia
   Adrenal insufficiency
   Hypopituitarism
   Diabetic ketoacidosis
Other systemic disorders (especially in the elderly coma-
      tose)
   Pancreatitis
   Uremia
   Hepatic failure
   Congestive heart failure
   Myocardial infarction
   Respiratory failure
   Gambian sleeping sickness
Drugs
   Ethanol
   Barbiturates
   Sedatives
   Phenothiazines
   General anesthesia
Hypothalamic and central nervous system dysfunction (hy-
      pothermia may be paroxysmal)
   Wernicke's encephalopathy
   Seizure
   Cerebrovascular accidents, paralysis, paresis

Head trauma
Brain tumors
Spinal cord transection above T1
Anorexia nervosa
Shapiro's syndrome
Agenesis of the corpus callosum
Spontaneous periodic hypothermia
Other hypothalamic lesions (e.g., sarcoidosis, infarction, or midbrain lesions)
Dermal disorders
  Burns
  Erythrodermas
Sepsis
Protein-calorie malnutrition
Iatrogenic causes
  Administration of cold blood or IV fluids
  Iced saline gastric lavage
  Peritoneal dialysis

References

1. Reuler JB: Hypothermia: Pathophysiology, Clinical Settings, and Management. *Ann Intern Med* 89:519, 1978.
2. Fitzgerald FR, Jessop C: Accidental Hypothermia: A Report of 22 Cases and Review of the Literature. *Adv Intern Med* 27:127, 1982.
3. Petersdorf RG: Hypothermia and Hyperthermia. In general reference 1, pp 2194–2200.

4-E. Weight Gain

Increased body fluid (see 2-B)
Exogenous obesity
Cushing's syndrome
Hypogonadism
Hyperprolactinemia
Hypothyroidism
Insulinoma
Congenital diseases
   Pseudohypoparathyroidism
   Prader-Willi syndrome
   Börjeson syndrome
   Alström syndrome
   Cohen syndrome
   Blount disease
   Laurence-Moon-Biedl syndrome
   Biemond syndrome
   Carpenter syndrome
Drugs
   Oral contraceptive use
   Pharmacologic doses of glucocorticoids
Disturbances of hypothalamic satiety centers
   Tumors
   Trauma
   Encephalitis
Acromegaly

Reference
1. Foster DW: Eating Disorders: Obesity, Anorexia Nervosa
   and Bulimia Nervosa. In general reference 9, p 1352.

4-F. Weight Loss

Endocrine disorders
    Diabetes mellitus (untreated or poorly treated)
    Diabetic neuropathic cachexia
    Thyrotoxicosis
    Adrenal insufficiency
    Pheochromocytoma
    Panhypopituitarism
Gastrointestinal disease
    Decreased food intake/malnutrition
        Poor or absent teeth
        Oral disease
    Esophageal disease
        Reflux
        Esophagitis
        Stricture
        Neoplasm
        Neuromuscular dysfunction
    Obstruction secondary to chronic peptic ulcer
    Abdominal angina
    Maldigestion/malabsorption (see 6-G)
    Inflammatory bowel disease
    Pernicious anemia
    Post-antrectomy (especially Billroth II)
Infection, especially:
    HIV
    Parasitic infestation
    Mycobacterium avium pulmonary infections
    Bacterial endocarditis
    Fungal diseases
    Amebic abscess
    Visceral leishmaniasis
    Giardiasis
    Cryptosporidiosis
    Chronic pleuropulmonary suppurative disease (e.g., empyema)
    Ankylosing spondylitis
    Thiamine deficiency
Malignancy, especially:
    Gastrointestinal
    Pancreatic
    Pulmonary
    Hepatic
    Biliary
    Leukemia
    Lymphoma

Somatostatinoma
Glucagonoma
Myelofibrosis
Psychiatric disease
Anorexia nervosa
Conversion disorders
Depression
Psychosis
Schizophrenia
Anxiety
Severe chronic organ failure
Renal failure
Heart failure (cardiac cachexia)
Pulmonary disease
Hepatic disease
Systemic lupus erythematosus

Reference
1. Foster DW: Gain and Loss In Weight. In general reference 1, p 260.

4-G. Adrenal Insufficiency

Primary
Idiopathic/autoimmune
Tuberculosis
Vascular
Hemorrhage
Sepsis
Hypotension
Anticoagulants
Interleukin-2 therapy
Coagulopathy
Trauma
Surgery
Pregnancy
Neonatal
Waterhouse-Friderichsen syndrome
Infarction
Thrombosis
Post-adrenal venography
Embolism
Arteritis
Infection
Fungal

Histoplasmosis
Coccidioidomycosis
Paracoccidioidomycosis
Blastomycosis
Moniliasis
Torulopsosis
Cryptococcosis
Syphilis
AIDS
  Cytomegalovirus
  Mycobacterium avium
  Cryptococcus
  Metastatic Kaposi's sarcoma
Infiltrative
  Hemochromatosis
  Sarcoidosis
  Amyloidosis
Neoplastic
  Lymphoma
  Metastatic cancer
  Leukemic infiltration
Iatrogenic
  Irradiation
  Bilateral adrenalectomy
Drugs (especially in those with limited adrenal reserve)
  Metyrapone
  Aminoglutethimide
  Trilostane
  Ketoconazole
  Rifampin
  Etomidate
  Suramin
  Phenytoin
  Barbiturates
  o,p'-DDD
  Spironolactone
Congenital/genetic
  Adrenoleukodystrophy/adrenomyelodystrophy
  Congenital adrenal hyperplasia
  Adrenal hypoplasia/aplasia
  Familial glucocorticoid deficiency (hereditary unrespon-
    siveness to adrenocorticotropic hormone [ACTH])
Defective cholesterol mechanism

Secondary (Pituitary) or Tertiary (Hypothalamic)
Pituitary/hypothalamic lesions (see 4-Q)
Isolated ACTH deficiency

Glucocorticoid therapy withdrawal
Following removal of cortisol-secreting adrenal tumor

References
1. Orth DN, Kovacs WJ, Debold CR: The Adrenal Cortex. In general reference 9, pp 525–529.
2. Williams GH, Dluhy RG: Disorders of the Adrenal Cortex. In general reference 1, p 1729.

4-H. Diabetes Insipidus

Nephrogenic (see 7-B)
Central
    Idiopathic
        Familial
        Sporadic
    Traumatic
        Head injury (basilar skull fracture)
        Birth trauma
    Iatrogenic
        Surgery (hypophysectomy)
        Irradiation
    Infection
        Basilar meningitis
        Encephalitis
        Measles
        Mumps
        Diphtheria
        Scarlet fever
        Landry-Guillain-Barré syndrome
        Brain abscess
        Tuberculosis
        Brucellosis
        Actinomycosis
        Syphilis
        Blastomycosis
    Vascular
        Thrombotic thrombocytopenic purpura
        Pituitary apoplexy
        Sheehan's syndrome
        Hemorrhage
        Thrombosis
        Aneurysm
        Vasculitis
        Intraventricular hemorrhage

Sickle cell crisis
Shock
Cardiopulmonary arrest
Aortocoronary bypass
Neoplasm
   Glioma
   Craniopharyngioma
   Astrocytoma
   Dysgerminoma
   Pinealoma
   Meningioma
   Leukemia
   Large pituitary adenoma
   Lymphoma
   Metastatic cancer (especially breast and lung)
Infiltrative
   Amyloidosis
   Histiocytosis X
   Eosinophilic granuloma
   Sarcoidosis
   Wegener's granulomatosis
Miscellaneous
   Collagen vascular disease
   Fat embolus
   Suprasellar and intrasellar cysts
   Anorexia nervosa
   Empty-sella syndrome
   Wolfram (DIDMOAD [diabetes insipidus, diabetes mel-
      litus, optic atrophy, deafness]) syndrome
   Circulating antibodies to vasopressin-producing cells

References
1. Coe FL: Alterations in Urinary Function. In general reference 1, p 275.
2. Reeves WB, Andreoli TE: The Posterior Pituitary and
   Water Metabolism. In general reference 9, pp 333–334.
3. Moses AM, Notman DD: Diabetes Insipidus and SIADH.
   Adv Int Med 27:73, 1973.

4-I. Hyperglycemia

Inadequate dietary preparation for glucose tolerance test
Spontaneous diabetes mellitus
  Type I (insulin dependent)
  Type II (non–insulin dependent)
Secondary diabetes mellitus
  Pancreatic disease
    Acute, chronic, or recurrent pancreatitis
    Pancreatectomy
    Pancreatic carcinoma
    Hemochromatosis
    Cystic fibrosis
    Malnutrition-related diabetes mellitus
  Hormonal abnormalities
    Increased counterregulatory hormones due to stress
      Infection
      Myocardial infarction
      Stroke
      Renal insufficiency
      Hepatic insufficiency
    Acromegaly
    Cushing's syndrome
    Hyperprolactinemia
    Carcinoid syndrome
    Primary aldosteronism
    Pheochromocytoma
    Glucagonoma
    Somatostatinoma
    VIPoma
    Hyperthyroidism
  Drug-induced
    Asparaginase
    Glucocorticoids and ACTH
    Estrogens, including oral contraceptives
    Thiazides and (less well-substantiated) loop diuretics
    Phenytoin
    Octreotide
    Salicylates
    Nicotinic acid
    Sympathomimetic agents
    Chlorpromazine
    Oxymethalone
    Danazol
    Diazoxide
    Growth hormone
    Pentamidine

Vacor
Indomethacin
Antiinsulin receptor antibodies
Insulin receptor abnormalities
Syndromes with increased risk of hyperglycemia
  Down's syndrome
  Turner's syndrome
  Alström's syndrome
  Laurence-Moon-Biedl syndrome
  Prader-Willi syndrome
  Werner's syndrome
  Cockayne's syndrome
  Ataxia-telangiectasia
  Myotonic dystrophy
  Panhypopituitary dwarfism
  Rabson-Mendenhall syndrome
  Leprechaunism
  Lipodystrophic syndromes
  Wolfram (DIDMOAD) syndrome
  Freidreich's ataxia
  Huntington's chorea
  Type I glycogen storage disease
  Acute intermittent porphyria
  Hermann's syndrome
  Klinefelter's syndrome
  Isolated growth hormone deficiency
  Machado disease
  Impaired glucose tolerance
  Gestational diabetes
  Mutant insulins (e.g., insulin Chicago)

Factors Causing Worsening of Compensated Diabetes (see also 3-I)
Increased caloric intake
Weight gain
Decreased exercise
Infection
Trauma
Surgery
Stroke
Pregnancy
Myocardial infarction
Drugs (see above)

Reference
1. Kahn CR, Catanese VM: Secondary Forms of Diabetes Mellitus. In general reference 8, pp 1087–1093.

4-J. Hypoglycemia

Fasting
Overutilization of glucose
  Prolonged exercise
  Insulin excess
    Pancreatic beta-cell disorders
      Insulinoma
      Islet-cell hyperplasia
      Nesidioblastosis
      Adenomatosis
      Beckwith's syndrome
      Leprechaunism
     Neonatal hypoglycemia (diabetic mother)
     Erythroblastosis fetalis
    Extrapancreatic tumors
      Bulky mesenchymal tumors
      Hepatomas
      Adrenocortical carcinomas
      Mesotheliomas
      Gastrointestinal carcinomas
      Lymphomas/leukemias
      Other (kidney, ovary, lung)
  Systemic carnitine deficiency
  Sepsis
  Deficiency in enzymes of fat oxidation
  HMG CoA lyase deficiency
  Maple syrup urine disease
  Antiinsulin antibodies
  Antiinsulin receptor antibodies
  Drug-induced overutilization
    Insulin (iatrogenic or factitious)
    Sulfonylureas, phenformin, metformin (iatrogenic or
      factitious)
Underproduction of glucose
  Inborn errors of glycogen metabolism
  Disorders of gluconeogenesis
  Severe hepatic dysfunction
  Congestive heart failure
  Falciparum malaria (children)
  Deficiencies of insulin counterregulatory hormones
    Growth hormone deficiency (children)
    Adrenal insufficiency
    Adrenal hyporesponsiveness of small-for-gestational-
      age (SGA) babies
    Glucagon deficiency

Hypothyroidism
Epinephrine deficiency (infants)
Hypopituitarism
Uremia
Substrate deficiency
Fasting hypoglycemia of pregnancy (late)
Ketotic hypoglycemia of infancy
Severe malnutrition
Ackee fruit ingestion
Idiopathic hypoglycemia of infancy and childhood
Drug-induced hypoglycemia
Salicylates
Ethanol
Pentamidine
Sulfonamides
Chloramphenicol
Oxytetracycline
Phenylbutazone
Coumarin derivatives
Probenecid
Haloperidol
Chlorpromazine
Anabolic steroids
Monoamine oxidase inhibitors
Encainide
Acetaminophen
Acetazolamide
Beta receptor blocking drugs
Aluminum hydroxide
Chloroquine
Cimetidine
Diphenhydramine
Disopyramide
Doxepin
EDTA
Fenoterol
Mesoxylate
Tris(hydroxymethyl)aminomethane (TRIS)
Isoproterenol
Mebendazole
Ouabain
Perhexilin
Hypoglycins
Terbutaline
Sulfadiazine
Ritodrino
Ranitidine

Quinine (IV)
Propoxyphene
Potassium para-aminobenzoate
Phenindione
Paraaminosalicylic acid
Orphenadrine
Lithium
Lidocaine
Isoxsuprine
Indomethacin
Imipramine
Clofibrate (potentiates oral agents)
Guanethidine
Tranylcypromine

Reactive
Induced by glucose
  Alimentary
    Partial or total gastrectomy
    Rapid gastric emptying
    Thyrotoxicosis
    Pyloroplasty
    Gastrojejunostomy
    Peptic ulcer disease
  Functional/idiopathic/spontaneous reactive hypoglycemia
  Early type II diabetes mellitus
  Endocrine deficiencies
    Adrenal insufficiency
    Hypothyroidism
  Discontinuation of total parenteral nutrition
Induced by other substrates
  Galactosemia
  Leucine-induced hypoglycemia
  Ethanol

References
1. Cryer PE: Glucose Homeostasis and Hypoglycemia. In general reference 9, p 1234.
2. Foster DW, Rubenstein AH: Hypoglycemia. In general reference 1, pp 1760–1764.
3. Lefèbvre PJ, Scheen AJ: Hypoglycemia. In Rifkin H, Porte D (eds): *Ellenberg and Rifkin's Diabetes Mellitus.* New York: Elsevier, 1990, pp 896–904.

4-K. Hyperlipidemias

Type I (chylomicrons)
  Primary
    Familial lipoprotein lipase deficiency
    Familial apolipoprotein C-II deficiency
    Inherited circulating lipoprotein inhibitor
  Secondary
    Dysglobulinemias (lupus, myeloma, lymphoma, Waldenström's)
    Severe untreated diabetes mellitus
    High-dose glucocorticoids
    Glycogen storage disease
Type IIA (low-density lipoproteins [LDL]) and IIB (LDL + very low-density lipoproteins [VLDL])
  Primary
    Familial hypercholesterolemia
      Deficiency of LDL receptors
      Defective LDL receptors
      LDL internalization defect
    Familial combined hyperlipidemia
  Secondary
    IIA and IIB
      Nephrotic syndrome
      Biliary obstruction
      Pregnancy
      Hypothyroidism
      Glucocorticoids (low-dose)
      Cushing's syndrome
      Werner's syndrome
    IIA only
      Liver disease (lipoprotein X)
      Excess dietary cholesterol
      Acute intermittent porphyria
      Anorexia nervosa
      Dysglobulinemias
    IIB only
      Diabetes mellitus (moderate)
Type III (intermediate-density lipoproteins)
  Primary
    Apolipoprotein E2 homozygotes
    Other apolipoprotein E variants
    Apolipoprotein E deficiency
    Hepatic lipase deficiency
  Secondary
    Hypothyroidism
    Diabetes mellitus (moderate)

      Beta blockers
      Thiazides
      Uremia
      Dysglobulinemias
Type IV (VLDL)
  Primary
    Familial hypertriglyceridemia
    Familial combined hyperlipidemia
    Sporadic hypertriglyceridemia
  Secondary
    Alcohol
    Nephrotic syndrome
    Diabetes mellitus (moderate)
    Hypothyroidism
    Pancreatitis
    Uremia
    Glucocorticoids (low-dose)
    Cushing's syndrome
    Estrogen or oral contraceptive therapy
    Type I glycogenosis
    Isotretinoin therapy
    Obesity
    Pregnancy
    Stress
    Thiazides
    Beta-adrenergic blockers
    Acromegaly
    Lipodystrophy (congenital or acquired)
    Hypopituitarism (ateliotic dwarfism)
Type V (VLDL and chylomicrons)
  Primary
    Familial hypertriglyceridemia (severe form)
    Familial lipoprotein lipase deficiency
    Familial combined hyperlipidemia (rarely)
    Familial apolipoprotein C-11 deficiency
  Secondary
    Diabetes mellitus (moderate or severe)
    Lipodystrophy (congenital or acquired)
    Estrogen or oral contraceptive therapy
    Pregnancy
    Alcohol
    Uremia
    Nephrotic syndrome
    Dysglobulinemias
    Hypothyroidism
    High-dose glucocorticoids
    Glycogen storage disease

Hypopituitarism (ateliotic dwarfism)
Isotretinoin therapy

References
1. Schaefer EJ, Levy RI: Pathogenesis and Management of Lipoprotein Disorders. *N Engl J Med* 312:1300, 1985.
2. Bierman EL, Glomset JA: Disorders of Lipid Metabolism. In general reference 9, p 1367.

4-L. Goiter

Diffuse Goiter
Euthyroid or hypothyroid
  Nontoxic diffuse goiter
    Intrinsic growth potential
    Thyroid growth-stimulating immunoglobulins
    Thyroid-stimulating hormone (TSH)
    Other growth factors
    Thyroiditis
      Hashimoto's thyroiditis
      Subacute (DeQuervain's, granulomatous) thyroiditis
      Painless (silent) thyroiditis
      Acute (suppurative) thyroiditis
      Riedel's syndrome
      Sarcoidosis
  Defects in hormone synthesis (dyshormonogenesis)
  Iodine deficiency
  Amyloidosis
  Ingestion of goitrogens
    Drugs
      Resorcinol
      Paraaminobenzoic acid
      Thiocyanate and isothiocyanate
      Perchlorate
      Antithyroid agents
        Propylthiouracil
        Methimazole
        Carbimazole
        Neonatal from maternal antithyroid therapy or iodine
      Sulfonamides
      p-Aminosalicylic acid
      Flavanoids
      Disulfides

Phenolic and phthalate ester derivatives
  Pyridines
  Polychlorinated and polybrominated biphenyls
  Other organochlorines
  Polycyclic aromatic hydrocarbons
  Ethionamide
  Dimercaprol
  Sulfonylureas
Amphenone
Aminoglutethimide
Phenylbutazone
Iodides
Amiodarone
Lithium carbonate
Cobalt
Goitrin
Brassica genus (cabbage, turnips, brussel sprouts, rutabagas)
Cyanaglucosides (cassava, maize, bamboo shoots, sweet potatoes, lima beans)
Soybean milk/soybean flour
Generalized resistance to thyroid hormone (GRTH)
Hyperthyroid
  Graves' disease
  Subacute thyroiditis
  Painless (silent) thyroiditis
  "Hashitoxicosis"
  Neonatal (mother with Graves' disease)
  Inappropriate thyroid-stimulating hormone secretion (rare)
    Ectopic
    Pituitary
      Tumor
      Isolated pituitary resistance to thyroid hormone (PRTH)

Multinodular Goiter
Nontoxic nodular goiter (see Diffuse Goiter: Euthyroid or hypothyroid)
Multiple adenomas
Toxic multinodular goiter

References
1. Davis PJ, Davis FB: Nontoxic Goiter. In general reference 8, pp 306–308.
2. Larsen PR, Ingbar SH: The Thyroid Gland. In general reference 9, pp 455–459.

4-M. Solitary Thyroid Nodule

Benign adenoma (may be functional or nonfunctional)
  Macrofollicular (simple colloid)
  Microfollicular (fetal)
  Embryonal (trabecular)
  Hürthle cell
  Atypical
  Adenoma with papillae
  Signet-ring adenomas
Malignancy
  Papillary carcinoma
  Mixed papillary-follicular carcinoma
  Follicular carcinoma
  Lymphoma
  Medullary carcinoma
  Anaplastic carcinoma
  Sarcoma
  Metastases to the thyroid
Thyroiditis
  Hashimoto's thyroiditis
  Subacute thyroiditis
  Acute (suppurative) thyroiditis
  Pneumocystis carinii infection (in AIDS)
  Riedel's struma
Simple cysts
Miscellaneous
  Hematoma
  Thyroid lobulation
  Granulomatous disease (e.g., sarcoidosis)
  Clinically inapparent multinodular goiter
  Unilateral lobes
  Agenesis or following hemithyroidectomy
Nonthyroid lesions
  Thyroglossal duct cyst
  Lymph node
  Carotid aneurysm
  Parathyroid cyst
  Parathyroid adenoma
  Laryngocele/bronchocele
  Cystic hygroma
  Lipoma
  Dermoid
  Teratoma

References
1. Mazzaferri EL: Management of a Solitary Thyroid Nodule. *N Engl J Med* 328:553, 1993.
2. Ahmann AJ, Wartofsky L: The Thyroid Nodule. In general reference 8, p 313.

4-N. Thyrotoxicosis

Thyrotoxicosis with hyperthyroidism (high or normal radioactive iodine uptake)
  Intrinsic thyroid autonomy
    Toxic adenoma
    Toxic multinodular goiter
  Abnormal thyroid stimulator
    Graves' disease
    Neonate of mother with Graves' disease
    Tumors secreting excessive human chorionic gonadotropin (HCG)
      Choriocarcinoma
      Hydatidiform mole
      Embryonal cell carcinoma of testis
    Hashitoxicosis
  Inappropriate thyroid-stimulating hormone (TSH) secretion
    Pituitary adenoma
    Isolated pituitary resistance to thyroid hormone (PRTH)
Thyrotoxicosis without hyperthyroidism (low radioactive iodine uptake)
  Inflammatory diseases
    Subacute thyroiditis
    Painless ("silent") thyroiditis
  Extrathyroidal source of hormone
    Hormone ingestion
      Iatrogenic
      Thyrotoxicosis factitia
      "Hamburger" thyrotoxicosis
    Ectopic thyroid tissue
      Metastatic differentiated thyroid cancer
      Struma ovarii
Hyperthyroidism with low radioactive iodine uptake
  Iodine-induced thyrotoxicosis (Jod-Basedow)

References
1. Burman KD: Hyperthyroidism. In general reference 8, pp 335–340.

2. Wartofsky L, Ingbar SH: Diseases of the Thyroid. In general reference 1, pp. 1702–1708.

4-O. Hypothyroidism

Primary hypothyroidism
  Thyroid agenesis or hypoplasia
  Destruction of gland
    Surgical removal
    Radioactive iodine therapy
    External irradiation for nonthyroid malignancies
    Thyroid growth blocking antibodies
    Interleukin-2 therapy
    Lymphokine-activated killer (LAK) cell therapy
    Replacement of thyroid tissue
      Thyroid cancer
      Cystinosis
      Metastatic nonthyroid cancer
      Riedel's struma
      Lymphoma
      Sarcoidosis and other granulomatous diseases
      Scleroderma
      Amyloidosis
      Hemochromatosis
    Pan-thyroiditis
      Acute thyroiditis (bacterial, mycobacterial, fungal, parasitic, gummatous)
      Pneumocystis carinii infection (in AIDS)
      Painless thyroiditis
      Subacute thyroiditis
      Hashimoto's thyroiditis
    Idiopathic atrophy (?autoimmune)
  TSH receptor abnormalities
  Inhibition of thyroid hormone synthesis
    Iodine deficiency
    Inherited enzyme defects (dyshormonogenesis)
    Drugs and goitrogens (see 4-L, Ingestion of Goitrogens)
      Addition of bile acid sequestrants to levothyroxine therapy
      Addition of sucralfate to levothyroxine therapy
    Addison's disease (reversible hypothyroidism)
    Selenium deficiency

Transient
  After surgery or radioactive iodine
  Postpartum thyroiditis
  Subacute thyroiditis
  Silent (painless) thyroiditis
Generalized resistance to hormone therapy
Secondary (pituitary) or tertiary (hypothalamic)—see 4-Q

References
1. Larsen PR, Ingbar SH: The Thyroid Gland. In general reference 9, pp 453–459.
2. Wartofsky L, Ingbar SH: Diseases of the Thyroid. In general reference 1, pp 1699–1702.

4-P. Serum Thyroxine

Elevated
  Thyrotoxicosis (see 4-N)
  Therapy with thyroxine (L-thyroxine or D-thyroxine)
  Elevated levels of serum thyroid-binding proteins
    Estrogens (endogenous or exogenous)
      Pregnancy
      Estrogen-containing medications (including oral contraceptives)
      Estrogen-secreting tumors
    Clofibrate
    Heroin
    Methadone
    Progestins
    Fluorouracil
    Propranolol
    Amphetamines (transient)
    Biliary cirrhosis
    Increased T_4 binding to variant albumins or thyroxine-binding prealbumins
    Acute and chronic active hepatitis
    Neonatal state
    Perphenazine/phenothiazines
    Genetically increased thyroxine-binding globulin
  Familial dysalbuminemic hyperthyroxinemia
  Acute intermittent porphyria
  Endogenous anti-T_4 antibodies
  Human antimouse antibodies
  Generalized resistance to thyroid hormone (GRTH)

Inhibition of T_4 to T_3 conversion
    Drugs (amiodarone, iopanoic acid, sodium ipodate)
    5'deiodinase deficiency
    Nonthyroidal illness
    Acute psychiatric illness
    Amphetamine use
    Nonequilibrium conditions
    T_4 replacement of hypothyroid patients
    Neonatal period
Decreased
  Hypothyroidism (primary or secondary) (see 4-O)
  Decreased levels of serum thyroid-binding proteins
    Protein loss (e.g., nephrotic syndrome)
    Severe systemic illness
    Genetically decreased thyroxine-binding globulin
    Androgens and anabolic steroids
    Aspirin
    Chlorpropamide
    Sulfonamides
    Asparaginase
  Displacement of T_4 from binding sites
    Halofenate
    Heparin (acutely)
    Phenylbutazone
    Phenytoin
    Tolbutamide
    Penicillin
  Increased T_4 hepatic metabolism
    Chlorpromazine
    Phenytoin
    Carbamazepine
    Phenobarbital
    Reserpine
    Rifampin
  Chronic liver disease
  Acromegaly
  Glucocorticoid excess or ACTH therapy
  Severe acidosis
  Testosterone-producing tumors
  Nonthyroidal illness
  Therapy with T_3 alone

References

1. Wallach J: *Interpretation of Diagnostic Tests* (5th ed).
   Boston: Little, Brown, 1992, pp 447–448.
2. Ingbar SH. The Thyroid Gland. In general reference 9,
   p 696.

4-Q. Pituitary/Hypothalamic Lesions

Invasive
  Craniopharyngioma
  Pituitary adenoma
  Rathke's pouch cyst
  Meningioma
  Aneurysm
  Arteriovenous anomalies
  Metastatic tumor
  Optic glioma
  Hamartoma
  Sarcoma
  Teratoma
  Ectopic pinealoma
  Leukemia
  Lymphoma
  Chordoma
Ischemic
  Sheehan's syndrome
  Diabetes mellitus
  Sickle cell anemia
  Collagen vascular disease
  Temporal arteritis
Infiltrative
  Hemochromatosis
  Sarcoidosis
  Amyloidosis
  Histiocytosis X
  Wegener's granulomatosis
  Tay-Sachs disease
Injury
  Basilar skull fracture
  Acute epidural and subdural hematoma
  Post–traumatic chronic brain syndrome
  Subarachnoid hemorrhage
Infectious
  Tuberculosis
  Meningitis
  Leukemia
  Fungal infections
  Encephalitis
  Syphilis
  Brucellosis
Immunologic
  Lymphocytic hypophysitis

Iatrogenic
  Surgery (hypophysectomy)
  Radiation therapy
  Immunosuppressive drugs
Idiopathic
Isolated
  Isolated growth hormone deficiency
  Isolated vasopressin deficiency
  Isolated adrenocorticotropic hormone (ACTH) deficiency
  Isolated thyroid-stimulating hormone (TSH) deficiency
  Isolated prolactin deficiency
  Kallmann's syndrome (hypothalamic hypogonadotropic
    hypogonadism)
  Acute intermittent porphyria
  Anencephaly

Reference

1. Findling JW, Tyrrell JB: Anterior Pituitary Gland. In
Greenspan FS (ed): *Basic and Clinical Endocrinology*.
Norwalk: Appleton & Lange, 1991, p 106.

4-R. Male Hypogonadism

Primary
  Developmental
    Klinefelter's syndrome
    XX Male
    XYY Syndrome
    Defective hormone synthesis or action
      Male pseudohermaphroditism
      Reifenstein's syndrome
      5α-Reductase deficiency
    Congenital anorchia
    Myotonic dystrophy
    Pseudo-Turner's syndrome (Noonan's syndrome)
    Sertoli-cell–only syndrome
Acquired
  Viral orchitis
  Trauma
  Radiation
  Drugs
    Spironolactone
    Alcohol

Marijuana
Cyclophosphamide
Autoimmune destruction
Granulomatous disease
Adult seminiferous tubule failure
Secondary or tertiary
Hypopituitarism (see 4-Q)
Cushing's syndrome
Hyperprolactinemia
Pituitary dwarfism
Constitutional delay of puberty
Severe illness (acute or chronic)
Kallman's syndrome
Laurence-Moon-Biedl syndrome
Prader-Willi syndrome
Fröhlich's syndrome
Isolated luteinizing hormone (LH) deficiency (fertile
    eunuch syndrome)

Reference

1. Grumbach MM, Styne DM: Puberty: Ontogeny, Neuro-
   endocrinology, Physiology, and Disorders. In general
   reference 9, 1171–1183.

4-S. Impotence

Neurologic
Amyotrophic lateral sclerosis
Arachnoiditis
Friedreich's ataxia
General paresis
Head injury
Herniated disk
Hypothalamic disease
Pelvic/retroperitoneal lymphadenopathy
Multiple sclerosis
Peripheral neuropathy
Pernicious anemia
Spina bifida
Spinal cord transection/injury
Spinal cord tumor
Spinal cord syrinx
Subacute combined degeneration

Sympathectomy
Tabes dorsalis
Temporal lobe disorders
Transverse myelitis
Endocrine
  Diabetes mellitus
  Hypopituitarism (see 4-Q)
  Hyperprolactinemia
  Cushing's syndrome
  Feminizing testicular or adrenal tumor
  Hypogonadism (see 4-R)
  Hypothyroidism
  Thyrotoxicosis
Psychogenic
Vascular
  Aneurysm
  Aortoiliac arteriosclerosis
  Arteritis
  Leriche's syndrome
  Embolism
  Priapism
  Thrombosis
Drug-induced
  Central nervous system depressants
    Reserpine
    Clonidine
    Alpha-methyldopa
    Ethanol
    Barbiturates
    Benzodiazepines
    Phenothiazines
    Butyrophenones
    Phenytoin
    Primidone
    Carbamazepine
    Heroin
    Methadone
    Morphine
  Anticholinergic
    Atropine
    Ganglionic blocking agents
    Tricyclic antidepressants
    Disopyramide
  Antiadrenergic
    Guanethidine
    Benzhexol
    Benztropine

Propranolol
Prazosin
Phenoxybenzamine
Phentolamine
Thioridazine
Bethanidine
Debrisoquin
Antiandrogen
  Cyproterone acetate
  Spironolactone
  Cimetidine
  Estrogens
  Progestins
Others
  Amphetamines
  Monoamine oxidase inhibitors
  Cocaine
  Marijuana
Genitourinary
  Hypospadias
  Micropenis, other congenital deformities
  Pelvic fracture
  Penectomy
  Penile trauma
  Peyronie's disease
  Systemic sclerosis
  Phimosis
  Prostate irradiation
  Prostatitis
  Urethritis
  Seminal vesiculitis
  Cystitis
  Urethral stricture
  Hydrocele
  Genital malignancy
  Ruptured urethra
Surgical
  Perineal prostatic biopsy
  Perineal prostatectomy
  Abdominal-perineal resection
  Vascular surgery (abdominal aortic aneurysm repair)
  External sphincterotomy
Endurance factors
  Post–myocardial infarction
  Pulmonary insufficiency
  Anemia
  Systemic illnesses

Uremia
Hepatic failure
Sleep disorders

References
1. Cunningham GR, Karacan I: Impotence. In general reference 8, p 977.
2. Krane RJ, Goldstein I, DeTejada IS: Impotence. *N Engl J Med* 321:1648, 1989.

5 EYE

5-A. Eye Pain

Foreign-Body Sensation
Foreign body on cornea, conjunctiva, or eyelid
Ingrown lashes, entropion
Corneal inflammation, abrasion, blebs, dystrophies

Burning Pain
Refractive error, uncorrected
Exposure to irritants (e.g., wind, dust, cosmetics)
Conjunctivitis
Insufficient secretions (e.g., Sjögren's syndrome)
Corneal inflammation (keratitis)
    Infection
    Allergic blepharitis
    Trauma
    X-rays, ultraviolet light
    Associated with skin disease (e.g., psoriasis, erythema
      multiforme)

Aching, Boring Pain
Uveitis
Orbital periostitis, abscess
Herpes zoster infection

Retrobulbar neuritis
Tic douloureux
Aneurysm (e.g., circle of Willis)
Orbital neoplasm (primary or metastatic)

Tenderness, Pain on Pressure
Lid inflammation
Dacryocystitis, dacryoadenitis (inflammation of lacrimal sac
or gland)
Corneal foreign body, abrasion, ulcer
Conjunctivitis
Scleritis, episcleritis
Iritis, iridocyclitis
Orbital cellulitis, periostitis, or abscess
Glaucoma
Sinusitis
Fever
Headache

Reference
1. Scheie HG, Albert DM: *Textbook of Ophthalmology* (9th
ed). Philadelphia: Saunders, 1977, p 159.

5-B. Red Eye

Conjunctivitis
  Infection
    Bacterial
    Viral
    Chlamydial
    Spirochetal
    Fungal
  Drugs, especially:
    Local anesthetics
    Antibiotics (e.g., neomycin, sulfonamides, chloram-
      phenicol, tetracycline, erythromycin)
    Mydriatic and miotic drugs (e.g, atropine)
  Contact allergy (e.g., drugs, cosmetics)
  Vernal conjunctivitis
Ciliary injection
  Iritis, iridocyclitis (see 5-H)
  Acute narrow-angle glaucoma
  Corneal foreign body, abrasion, or ulceration
Chorioretinitis

Scleritis
Subconjunctival hemorrhage (traumatic or spontaneous)

Reference
1. Scheie HG, Albert DM: *Textbook of Ophthalmology* (9th ed). Philadelphia: Saunders, 1977, p 359.

5-C. Visual Loss or Impairment

Cornea
Corneal edema
Keratitis
  Viral infection (especially herpes)
  Congenital syphilis
  Behcet's syndrome
  Reiter's syndrome
  Stevens-Johnson syndrome
  Allergic reactions
  Drying of eyes secondary to coma
  Mucopolysaccharidoses
Crystal deposition (e.g., cystinosis)
Corneal dystrophies
Keratoconus
Trauma

Aqueous Humor
Glaucoma

Vitreous Humor
Opacification
Hemorrhage (e.g., associated with diabetes, trauma, sickle cell disease)

Uveal Tract
Inflammation (see 5-H)
Hemorrhagic disease
Tumor, primary or metastatic

Lens
Refractive errors
  Myopia, hyperopia, presbyopia, astigmatism
  Lens sclerosis
  Large changes in blood sugar (e.g., diabetes mellitus)

Opacification (cataract)
  Age
  Diabetes mellitus
  Radiation
  Drugs (e.g., steroids, chlorpromazine)
  Hypoparathyroidism
  Congenital or hereditary causes (e.g., myotonic dystrophy, Fabry's disease, congenital rubella)
Dislocation
  Marfan's syndrome
  Homocystinuria
Trauma

Retina
Degeneration
  Congenital or hereditary diseases (e.g., retinitis pigmentosa, Laurence-Moon-Biedl syndrome, pseudoxanthoma elasticum)
  Macular degeneration (hereditary or senile)
  Paget's disease
  Acromegaly
  Hyperphosphatemia
Vascular lesions
  Central retinal vein occlusion
    External compression
    Degenerative venous disease
    Diabetes mellitus
    Leukemia
    Sickle cell disease
    Trauma
    Inflammation, infection
  Central retinal artery occlusion
    Thrombus
    Embolus
    Spasm
    Temporal arteritis
  Carotid or basilar artery embolus or thrombosis
  Hemorrhage, especially:
    Diabetes mellitus
    Hypertension
    Severe anemia (e.g., sickle cell, massive blood loss)
    Thrombotic thrombocytopenic purpura, disseminated intravascular coagulation
Toxins, especially:
  Methanol
  Quinine
  Carbon bisulfide

Detachment
Retinitis or chorioretinitis
  Toxoplasmosis
  Histoplasmosis
  Sarcoidosis
  Lupus erythematosus
  Polyarteritis nodosa
  Tuberculosis
  Syphilis
  Cytomegalovirus infection
  Bacterial sepsis, endocarditis
Tumor

Central Nervous System

Optic nerve disease
  Optic neuritis, neuropathy, atrophy (see 5-E)
  Prolonged papilledema
  Optic nerve trauma
Optic chiasm lesion
  Tumor (especially pituitary tumor, meningioma, meta-
    static tumor)
  Sarcoidosis
  Aneurysm of circle of Willis
Cerebral lesion
  Calcarine tract (optic radiation)
  Parietal lobe(s)
  Temporal lobe(s)
  Occipital lobe(s)
  Cortical blindness
  Migraine (usually transient)
  Head injury
  Hysteria

References

1. Wray SH, Slamovits TL, Burde RM: Disturbances of Vision and Ocular Movements. In general reference 1,
   p 143.
2. General reference 10, p 143.
3. General reference 22, p 190.

5-D. Exophthalmos

Pseudoexophthalmos
    Unilateral ocular enlargement (e.g., trauma, myopia,
      glaucoma)*
Lid retraction
Extraocular muscle paralysis secondary to surgery or nerve
    injury*
Graves' disease
Orbital inflammation*
    Acute
      Cellulitis
      Abscess
      Periostitis
      Cavernous sinus thrombosis
    Chronic granulomatous ("pseudotumor")
      Sarcoidosis
      Tuberculosis
      Syphilis
Trauma*
    Orbital hemorrhage, hematoma
    Orbital fracture with air leak from sinus
Orbital tumor*
    Meningioma
    Dermoid
    Hemangioma
    Neuroblastoma
    Neurofibroma
    Optic nerve glioma
    Lymphoma, leukemic infiltrates
    Metastatic carcinoma
    Lacrimal gland tumor
    Rhabdomyosarcoma
    Pseudotumor
Reticuloendotheliosis (especially Hand-Schüller-Christian
    disease)
Systemic disease
    Accelerated hypertension
    Alcoholism
    Chronic obstructive pulmonary disease
    Uremia
    Cushing's syndrome
    Superior mediastinal obstruction
Paranasal sinus or nasopharyngeal tumor, infection, muco-
    cele
Orbital cyst*

Orbital varices (especially associated with trauma, arterio-
venous malformation, hemangioma)*
Orbital aneurysm (e.g., ophthalmic artery)*
Congenital (e.g., genetic, racial)

References
1. General reference 1, p 1704.
2. Grove AS: Evaluation of Exophthalmos. *N Engl J Med*
292:1005, 1975.

*Usually unilateral.

5-E. Optic Nerve Atrophy

Ocular diseases causing retinal degeneration (e.g., retinitis
pigmentosa, extensive chorioretinitis)
Optic neuritis (optic nerve inflammation)
  Demyelinating disease
    Multiple sclerosis
    Diffuse cerebral sclerosis
    Schilder's disease
    Acute disseminated encephalomyelitis
    Neuromyelitis optica (Devic's disease)
  Infection
    Intraocular (keratitis, chronic uveitis, endophthalmitis)
    Extraocular (orbital cellulitis, meningitis, encephalitis,
      brain abscess)
    Bacterial (e.g., *Haemophilus influenzae*)
    Spirochetal (e.g., syphilis)
    Mycobacterial (e.g., tuberculosis)
    Viral (e.g., herpes zoster, mumps, measles, rubella; or
      mumps, measles, or rubella vaccine)
    Fungal (e.g., *Cryptococcus*)
    Protozoal/helminthic (e.g., toxoplasmosis, toxocariasis)
    Guillain-Barré syndrome
Optic neuropathy
  Ischemic disease
    Arteriosclerosis, accelerated hypertension
    Collagen-vascular disease (e.g., lupus erythematosus,
      temporal arteritis, Behçet's syndrome, polyarteritis
      nodosa, Buerger's disease)
    Glaucoma
    Diabetes mellitus
    Sarcoidosis

    Hyperthyroidism
    Sickle cell disease
    Severe anemia
    Polycythemia vera
    Orbital radiation
Drugs, toxins
    Methanol
    Tobacco and/or alcohol
    Chloroquine
    Lead
    Arsenic
    Quinine
    Thallium
    Ethambutol
    Isoniazid
    Ergot
    Disulfiram
    Chloramphenicol
Nutritional deprivation (especially alcoholism, pellagra, beriberi, pernicious anemia)
Optic nerve trauma
Optic nerve tumor (e.g., optic nerve glioma, meningioma, metastatic carcinoma)
Prolonged papilledema (see 5-F)
Intracranial lesions affecting visual pathways (with or without papilledema)
Congenital and hereditary diseases (e.g., leukodystrophies, optic nerve hypoplasia)

References
1. General reference 22, p 190.
2. General reference 10, p 353.
3. General reference 11, p 2091.

5-F. Papilledema*

Pseudotumor cerebri
Intracranial tumor (especially subtentorial)
  Meningioma
  Metastatic tumor
  Hodgkin's disease
  Optic nerve tumor
  Leukemia with optic nerve infiltrates
Infection (meningitis, encephalitis, brain abscess), especially:
  Bacterial
  Viral
  Tuberculous
  Syphilitic
  Fungal (especially cryptococcal)
Subarachnoid hemorrhage
Intracranial trauma (e.g., subdural or epidural hematoma,
    intracranial hemorrhage)
Vascular disease (involving retinal vessels)
  Hypertensive encephalopathy
  Collagen-vascular disease (especially lupus erythematosus)
  Granulomatous angiitis, other arteritides
  Central retinal vein occlusion
  Cavernous sinus thrombosis
Drugs and toxins
  Methanol
  Vitamin A
  Lead
  Arsenic
  Lithium
  Thallium
  Cisplatin
  Tetracycline
  Corticosteroids
  Progestins
  Nalidixic acid
Metabolic diseases
  Diabetes mellitus
  Adrenal insufficiency
  Hyperthyroidism
  Hypoparathyroidism
Sarcoidosis
Respiratory insufficiency with carbon dioxide retention

Congenital and developmental malformation (especially congenital hydrocephalus, craniosynostosis, Arnold-Chiari malformation, aqueductal stenosis)

Optic Disk Blurring and/or Edema Without Increased Intracranial Pressure
Hyperopia
Medullated nerve fibers
Disk drusen
Orbital lesions (e.g., orbital hemangioma, perioptic meningioma)
Ocular hypotonia (e.g., traumatic or surgical)
Ocular inflammatory disorders, especially:
  Uveitis (see 5-H)
  Optic neuritis (see 5-E)
  Papillophlebitis

References
1. General reference 10, p 353.
2. General reference 11, p 2105.

*Optic disk swelling associated with increased intracranial pressure.

5-G. Pupillary Abnormalities

Miosis
Aging
Drugs (especially pilocarpine, morphine, physostigmine)
Corneal or conjunctival irritation
Iritis
Posterior synechiae (postinflammatory)
Pontine lesions
Meningitis, encephalitis
Cavernous sinus thrombosis
Neurosyphilis (Argyll Robertson pupil)
Congenital absence of dilator pupillae muscle

Mydriasis
Drugs, especially:
  Atropine
  Phenylephrine
  Isoproterenol
  Epinephrine
  Cocaine
Angle-closure glaucoma

Coma, especially due to:
  Alcohol intoxication
  Diabetes mellitus
  Uremia
  Postepilepsy
  Meningitis
  Midbrain lesions
Optic neuropathy or atrophy (see 5-E)
Intracranial neoplasm or aneurysm
Ocular trauma (especially with tear of iris sphincter muscle)
Orbital or cranial trauma
Orbital or choroidal tumor

Anisocoria

Local causes
  Mydriatic or miotic drugs
  Injury to iris (d)*
  Inflammation
    Keratitis (c)
    Iridocyclitis (d or c)
    Posterior synechiae (c)
  Angle-closure glaucoma (d)
  Ischemia of anterior ocular segment (e.g., resulting from
      internal carotid artery insufficiency) (d)
  Disease of iris (e.g., aniridia) (d)
  Unilateral blindness resulting from optic or retinal
      causes (d)
  Prosthetic eye
Sphincter pupillae muscle paralysis (d)
  Intracranial infection, especially:
    Syphilis
    Herpes zoster
    Tuberculosis
    Encephalitis, meningitis
    Botulism
    Diphtheria
  Intracranial neoplasm
  Cerebral aneurysm
  Cavernous sinus thrombosis
  Subdural, extradural hemorrhage
  Degenerative nervous system disease
  Toxic polyneuritis (especially alcohol, lead, arsenic)
  Diabetes mellitus
Dilator pupillae muscle paralysis (c) (see Horner's Syn-
      drome below)
Others
  Tabes dorsalis (c)
  Midbrain lesion (d)
  Adie's syndrome (d)

Horner's Syndrome

Peripheral causes; compression of or injury to cervical
      nerve roots, ganglia, or efferent sympathetic fibers
  Mediastinal tumor (especially bronchogenic carcinoma,
      metastatic tumor, Hodgkin's disease)
  Thyroid adenoma
  Neurofibromatosis
  Trauma (surgical or accidental)
  Internal carotid artery aneurysm
Central nervous system causes
  Posterior inferior cerebellar artery occlusion
  Multiple sclerosis
  Syringomyelia
  Brainstem or cervical cord tumor
  Spinal cord trauma
Congenital

Reference

1. General reference 10, p 274.

*(d) indicates the affected pupil is dilated; (c) indicates the affected
pupil is constricted.

5-H. Uveitis

Infection (local inflammation of orbit, cornea, conjunctiva;
      meningitis)
  Bacterial, especially:
    Staphylococcus aureus
    Proteus species
    Pseudomonas aeruginosa
    Bacillus subtilis
    Coliforms
    Neisseria gonorrhoeae
  Mycobacterial
    Tuberculosis
    Leprosy
  Spirochetal (syphilis)
  Viral, especially:
    Herpes simplex, herpes zoster
    Cytomegalovirus
    Variola
    Vaccinia
    Mononucleosis
    Lymphogranuloma venereum

Rickettsial (typhus)
Fungal (especially histoplasmosis)
Protozoan, especially:
   Toxoplasmosis
   Amebic dysentery
   Malaria
   Sleeping sickness
Hypersensitivity reaction (especially airborne allergens,
      foods, protein antigens)
Irritant or toxic gases
Trauma (especially sympathetic ophthalmia [following globe
      perforation], following lens rupture, retained foreign
      body)
Systemic disease
   Collagen-vascular disease
      Systemic lupus erythematosus
      Ankylosing spondylitis
      Juvenile rheumatoid arthritis
      Reiter's syndrome
      Behçet's syndrome
      Polyarteritis nodosa
      Wegener's granulomatosis
   Sarcoidosis
   Diabetes mellitus
Lens disease
   Hypermature cataract
   Retention of lens material after lens extraction
   Endophthalmitis phacoanaphylactica
Blindness with degenerative changes
Necrosis of intraocular tumor
Idiopathic

References

1. General reference 10, p 283.
2. General reference 11, p 1554.

6 GASTROINTESTINAL AND HEPATIC SYSTEMS

6-A. Nausea and Vomiting*

Gastrointestinal Disorders
Obstructive vomiting
  Any cause of bowel obstruction (see 6-I)
Nonobstructive vomiting
  Gastroenteritis
  Peptic ulcer disease
  Gastritis
  Pancreatitis
  Cholecystitis
  Gastroesophageal reflux
  Hepatitis
  Choledocholithiasis
  Biliary stricture
  Peritonitis
  Appendicitis
  Postvagotomy syndrome
  Diabetic gastroparesis
  Superior mesenteric artery (SMA) syndrome
  Prior gastrointestinal surgery
  Carcinoma: stomach, small intestine, pancreas, biliary tract
  Ischemic bowel disease
  Idiopathic intestinal pseudoobstruction

Food poisoning
Eosinophilic gastroenteritis
Pancreatic pseudocyst
Postoperative paralytic ileus
Electrolyte abnormality
Uremia
Heavy metal toxicity
Idiopathic ileus
CNS tumors
Psychiatric disorder, eating disorder

Systemic Disorders
Acute infections (especially in children)
Reye's syndrome
Severe pain
Acute myocardial infarction
Congestive heart failure
Radiation sickness
Scleroderma
Amyloidosis
Acquired immunodeficiency syndrome (AIDS)
Carcinomatosis

Central Nervous System Disorders
Increased intracranial pressure
   Trauma
   Neoplasm
   Meningitis, encephalitis
   Hydrocephalus
   Reye's syndrome
Vestibular or middle ear disease
   Motion sickness
   Menière's disease
   Eighth nerve tumor
   Infection
Eye disorders
   Glaucoma
   Refractive error
Migraine headache
Autonomic epilepsy

Endocrine and Metabolic Disorders
Diabetic ketoacidosis
Metabolic acidosis from other causes
Uremia

Hypercalcemia
Hyponatremia
Hypothyroidism
Adrenal insufficiency
Hyperthyroidism
Hyperparathyroidism

Genitourinary Disorders
Pyelonephritis
Obstructive uropathy
Renal calculi
Salpingitis
Endometritis, parametritis

Drugs and Poisons
Chemotherapeutic agents
Alcohol
Anticholinergic drugs
Digitalis
Aminophylline
Colchicine
Morphine and derivatives
Ergot alkaloids
Antiarrhythmic drugs
Estrogens, oral contraceptives
Carbon monoxide
Carbon tetrachloride
Heavy metals (e.g., arsenic, mercury)
Nonsteroidal antiinflammatory drugs (NSAIDs)
Potassium chloride

Miscellaneous
Pregnancy
Nausea and vomiting of pregnancy
  Hyperemesis gravidarum
Psychogenic
  Bulimia
  Anorexia nervosa
  Rumination
Alcohol, drug withdrawal
Trauma (duodenal hematoma)
Pneumatosis intestinalis
Endometriosis
Graft versus host disease
Systemic infection

Reference
1. Feldman M: Nausea and Vomiting. In general reference
   12, p 222.

*The causes of nausea and vomiting are innumerable: this list is not
intended to include them all. The important categories of disorders
with vomiting as a major symptom are listed, and several examples
of each are given.

6-B. Dysphagia, Odynophagia

Oropharyngeal Causes
Painful swallowing
  Pharyngitis
  Herpes stomatitis
  Monilial stomatitis
  Mumps
  Vincent's angina
  Abscess
    Retropharyngeal
    Peritonsillar
  Malignancy
  Acute thyroiditis
Upper esophageal sphincter (UES) dysfunction
  Hypertensive UES
  Hypotensive UES
  Abnormal UES relaxation
  Familial dysautonomia
Esophageal web
Cervical osteophyte
Zenker's diverticulum
Pharyngeal paralysis
  Poliomyelitis
  Syringomyelia
  Cerebrovascular accident
  Amyotrophic lateral sclerosis
  Multiple sclerosis
  Glossopharyngeal neuritis
Pharyngeal muscle weakness
  Myasthenia gravis
  Myotonic dystrophy
  Restricted muscular dystrophy
    Oculopharyngeal
    Laryngeal esophageal
  Amyloidosis

Scleroderma
Dermatomyositis
Hyperthyroidism
Hypothyroidism
Polymyositis
Fixation of larynx
  Laryngeal neoplasm
  Scarring (e.g., secondary to radiation, surgery)
Congenital abnormalities

Esophageal Causes
Neuromuscular (motility) disorders
  Primary
    Achalasia
    Diffuse esophageal spasm
    Nutcracker esophagus
    Hypertensive lower esophageal sphincter
    Nonspecific esophageal dysmotility
  Secondary
    Diabetic neuropathy
    Scleroderma
    Other connective tissue diseases
    Chagas' disease
    Chronic idiopathic intestinal pseudoobstruction
Luminal narrowing
  Esophageal
    Reflux esophagitis
    Peptic stricture
    Carcinoma
    Esophageal web (Plummer-Vinson syndrome)
    Traumatic, corrosive stricture
    Lower esophageal (Schatzki) ring
    Traction diverticulum
    Midesophageal diverticulum
    Benign tumors (submucosal)
    Epiphrenic diverticulum
    Paraesophageal hernia
    Carcinoma of gastric cardia
    Medication-induced esophagitis
  Extraesophageal, intrathoracic
    Lymph node enlargement (e.g., tuberculosis, malignancy)
    Thyromegaly (benign, malignant)
    Mediastinal disease
      Malignancy
      Tuberculosis
      Other inflammatory lesions

Pulmonary abscess
Empyema
Pericardial effusion
Vascular lesions
  Aortic aneurysm
  Anomalous right subclavian artery
Cervical osteophyte
Foreign body

References

1. Pope CE: Heartburn, Dysphagia, and Other Esophageal Symptoms. In general reference 12, p 200.
2. Pope CE et al: The Esophagus. In general reference 12, p 541.
3. Eastwood GL: Esophageal Disorders. In general reference 13, p 3.

6-C. Abdominal Pain*

Abdominal Disorders
Intraperitoneal
  Inflammatory disorders
    Peritoneum
      Peritonitis (chemical or bacterial; see 6-J)
      Subdiaphragmatic abscess
      Familial Mediterranean fever
    Hollow viscera
      Gastroenteritis
      Appendicitis
      Cholecystitis
      Peptic ulcer disease
      Gastritis
      Duodenitis
      Crohn's disease
      Colitis (idiopathic and infectious)
      Diverticulitis
      Meckel's diverticulum
    Solid viscera
      Pancreatitis (see 6-K)
      Hepatitis (see 6-O)
      Abscess (especially hepatic, splenic, pancreatic)
    Pelvic viscera
      Pelvic inflammatory disease
      Tuboovarian disease
      Mittelschmerz

            Endometritis
            Endometriosis
            Salpingitis
            Fitz-Hugh-Curtis syndrome
        Mesentery
            Mesenteric lymphadenitis
    Mechanical disorders
        Hollow viscera
            Intestinal obstruction
            Intussusception
            Biliary tract obstruction
        Solid viscera
            Acute capsular distention
                Acute splenomegaly
                Acute hepatomegaly (especially hepatitis, hepatic
                    congestion, Budd-Chiari syndrome)
        Pelvic viscera
            Ovarian cyst/torsion
            Ectopic pregnancy
        Mesentery
            Omental torsion
    Malignancy
        Pancreatic
            Gastric
            Hepatic, primary or metastatic
            Colonic
            Small intestinal
            Ovarian
            Uterine
        Vascular disorders
            Intraabdominal bleeding
            Ischemia
                Mesenteric artery insufficiency or thrombosis
                Infarction (especially liver, spleen)
                Omental ischemia
    Irritable bowel syndrome
Extraperitoneal
    Pyelonephritis
    Ureteral obstruction (especially stones, tumor)
    Aortic aneurysm
        Rupture
        Dissection
        Expansion
    Perinephric abscess
    Psoas abscess
    Prostatitis
    Seminal vesiculitis
    Epididymitis

Extraabdominal Disorders
Thoracic
  Lung
    Pneumonia
    Pulmonary infarction
    Pneumothorax
    Empyema
    Pleuritis
  Heart
    Myocardial ischemia or infarction
    Pericarditis
    Myocarditis, endocarditis
  Esophagus
    Esophagitis
    Esophageal spasm
    Esophageal rupture
Neurologic
  Radiculitis
    Herpes zoster
    Degenerative arthritis
    Herniated intervertebral disk
    Tumor
  Causalgia
  Tabes dorsalis
  Abdominal epilepsy
Hematologic
  Leukemia
  Lymphoma
  Sickle cell crisis
  Hemolytic anemia
  Henoch-Schönlein purpura
Abdominal wall
  Contusion
  Hematoma
  Tumor
Toxins
  Insect bites
  Snake venom
Metabolic disorders
  Uremia
  Diabetes (especially ketoacidosis)
  Addisonian crisis
  Porphyria
  Lead poisoning
  Hyperlipidemia
  Hereditary angioneurotic edema
Psychiatric disorders
  Depression

Anxiety disorders
Schizophrenia
Factitious abdominal pain
Other
Acute glaucoma

Reference
1. Way LW: Abdominal Pain. In general reference 12, p
   238.

*See also 6-D.

6-D. Characteristic Location of Abdominal Pain Associated with Various Diseases*

Diffuse
Gastroenteritis
Peritonitis
Pancreatitis
Leukemia
Sickle cell crisis
Early appendicitis (may be periumbilical)
Mesenteric adenitis
Mesenteric thrombosis
Abdominal aortic aneurysm
Intussusception
Colitis
Intestinal obstruction
Inflammatory bowel disease
Metabolic, toxic, bacterial causes

Epigastric
Peptic ulcer disease
Pancreatitis
Gastritis
Cholecystitis
Reflux esophagitis
Myocardial ischemia
Pericarditis
Abdominal wall hematoma

Right Upper Quadrant
Cholecystitis
Choledocholithiasis

Hepatitis
Hepatic metastases
Hepatic abscess
Hepatocellular carcinoma
Hepatomegaly resulting from congestive heart failure
Budd-Chiari syndrome (hepatic vein obstruction)
Peptic ulcer
Pancreatitis
Retrocecal appendicitis
Renal pain
Herpes zoster
Myocardial ischemia
Pericarditis
Pneumonia
Empyema
Pulmonary infarction
Pleuritis

Left Upper Quadrant
Gastritis
Peptic ulcer disease
Pancreatitis
Splenic
   Enlargement, rupture
   Infarction, aneurysm
Renal pain
Herpes zoster
Myocardial ischemia
Pericarditis
Pneumonia
Empyema
Pulmonary infarction
Pleuritis

Right Lower Quadrant
Appendicitis
Intestinal obstruction
Crohn's disease
Diverticulitis
Cholecystitis
Perforated ulcer
Leaking aortic aneurysm
Abdominal wall hematoma
Ectopic pregnancy
Ovarian cyst or torsion
Salpingitis
Mittelschmerz
Endometriosis

Ureteral colic
Renal pain
Seminal vesiculitis
Psoas abscess

Left Lower Quadrant
Diverticulitis
Intestinal obstruction
Colon cancer
Appendicitis
Gastritis
Leaking aortic aneurysm
Inflammatory bowel disease
Abdominal wall hematoma
Splenic distention
Ectopic pregnancy
Mittelschmerz
Ovarian cyst or torsion
Salpingitis
Endometriosis
Ureteral colic
Renal pain
Seminal vesiculitis
Psoas abscess
Irritable bowel syndrome

*Modified from Schwartz SI: Manifestations of Gastrointestinal Disease. In Schwartz SI, Shires GT, Spencer FC (eds): *Principles of Surgery* (5th ed). New York: McGraw-Hill, 1989, p 1061. Copyright 1989 by McGraw-Hill Book Company.

6-E. Constipation

Simple Constipation
Low-residue diet
Chronic laxative and/or enema abuse
Muscular weakness

Gastrointestinal Disorders
Colonic, extraluminal obstruction
  Tumors
  Chronic volvulus
  Hernias
  Rectal prolapse
  Ascites
  Pregnancy
  Adhesions
Colonic, luminal disorders
  Tumors (benign, malignant)
  Fecal impaction
  Diverticulitis
  Strictures
    Chronic ulcerative colitis
    Recurrent diverticulitis
    Carcinoma
    Chronic amebiasis
    Lymphogranuloma venereum
    Syphilis
    Tuberculosis
    Ischemic colitis
    Endometriosis
    Postsurgical
  Intussusception
  Corrosive enemas
Anorectal disorders
  Proctitis (especially ulcerative)
  Hemorrhoids
  Fissures and fistulas (e.g., Crohn's disease)
  Perianal abscess
  Rectal prolapse
  Stenosis
    Neoplastic
    Inflammatory (lymphogranuloma venereum [LGV],
      ulcerative proctitis)
    Postsurgical
  Descending perineum syndrome
  Rectocele

Abnormalities of muscle function
    Irritable bowel syndrome
    Diverticular disease
    Muscular dystrophies
    Familial visceral myopathy
    Likongo's syndrome (hindgut dysgenesis)

Neuromuscular Disorders
Spinal cord disorders (especially trauma, multiple sclerosis, cauda equina tumor)
Diabetic autonomic neuropathy
Muscular abnormality

Neurologic Disorders
Central
    Multiple sclerosis
    Spinal cord lesions
    Parkinson's disease
    Shy-Drager syndrome
    Trauma to nervi erigentes
    Cerebrovascular accident
    Psychosis
    Senile dementia
    Tumor
Peripheral
    Hirschprung's disease
    Chagas' disease
    Neurofibromatosis
    Ganglioneuromatosis
    Autonomic neuropathy
    Colonic pseudoobstruction
    Hypoganglionosis and hyperganglionosis
    Intestinal pseudoobstruction
    Multiple endocrine neoplasia type IIB

Endocrine and Metabolic Disorders
Diabetes mellitus
Hypothyroidism
Hyperparathyroidism
Other hypercalcemic states
Pheochromocytoma
Hypokalomia
Panhypopituitarism
Heavy metal poisoning
Uremia
Porphyria
Pregnancy

Glucagonoma
Pseudohypoparathyroidism

Collagen Vascular and Other Muscle Disorders
Systemic sclerosis
Amyloidosis
Dermatomyositis
Myotonic dystrophy

Drugs
Antacids
   Calcium carbonate
   Aluminum hydroxide
Opiates
Anticholinergics
Anticonvulsants
Tricyclic antidepressants
Ganglionic blockers
Phenothiazines
Diuretics
Ferrous sulfate
Antihypertensives
Barium sulfate
Bismuth compounds
Ion-exchange resins
Antispasmodics
Antidepressants
Antipsychotics
Calcium channel blockers
Calcium supplements
Sucralfate
Cholestyramine
Bismuth
Monoamine-oxidase (MAO) inhibitors
Analgesics
Vinca alkaloids

Reference
1. Devroede G: Constipation. In general reference 12, p
   331.

6-F. Diarrhea

Acute Diarrhea
Infectious
  Viral gastroenteritis
  Bacterial
    Invasive (e.g., *Shigella, Salmonella, Campylobacter,*
      invasive *Escherichia coli, Yersinia*)
    Toxigenic (e.g., *Staphylococcus, E. coli, Clostridia,*
      Vibrio species, toxic shock syndrome)
  Protozoal (e.g., amebiasis, giardiasis)
Acquired immunodeficiency syndrome (AIDS)
Stress-induced
Traveler's diarrhea
Food allergy (rare)
Dietary indiscretion (e.g., prunes, unripe fruit, rhubarb)
Excessive alcohol ingestion
Gastrointestinal disorders
  Partial bowel obstruction
  Diverticulitis
  Appendicitis
  Ischemic bowel disease
  Pseudomembranous colitis
  Initial attack of ulcerative colitis or Crohn's disease
Systemic disorders
  Uremia
  Carcinoid syndrome
  Endocrine disorders
    Thyrotoxicosis
    Addisonian crisis
Poisoning
  Heavy metals (especially arsenic, cadmium, mercury)
  Mushrooms
Drugs
  Laxatives
  Broad-spectrum antibiotics
  Magnesium-containing antacids/products
  Lactulose
  Colchicine
  Digitalis
  Iron
  Guanethidine
  Methyldopa
  Hydralazine
  Quinidine
  Sorbitol

Fructose
Mannitol
Bran/fiber
Acute exacerbation of chronic diarrhea

Chronic Diarrhea
Mucosal inflammation
Ulcerative colitis, proctitis
Crohn's disease
Amebic colitis
Radiation enterocolitis
Ischemic colitis
Pseudomembranous colitis
Diverticulitis
Parasitic infestation
Lymphocytic colitis
Chemotherapy-induced mucositis
Graft versus host disease
Decreased solute absorption (osmotic diarrhea)
Disaccharidase deficiency
Monosaccharide malabsorption
Postgastrectomy "dumping" syndrome
Congenital chloridorrhea
Malabsorption syndromes (see 6-G)
Maldigestion syndromes (see 6-G)
Secretory diarrhea
Zollinger-Ellison syndrome (gastrinoma)
Pancreatic cholera (VIPoma)
Carcinoid syndrome
Medullary carcinoma of the thyroid
Hydroxy fatty acid excretion
Bile salt malabsorption
Sympathetic tissue tumors (ganglioneuromas)
Food allergy
Villous adenoma
Carotid body tumor
Stimulant/laxative abuse
Chronic infections
Inflammatory bowel disease
Lymphocytic/collagenous colitis
Lymphoma
Pseudopancreatic cholera syndrome
Motor disorders
Irritable bowel syndrome
Neoplasm (obstruction)
Postvagotomy
Postsurgical
Gastrectomy

Gastroenterostomy
Pyloroplasty
Gastroileal or gastrocolonic fistula

Miscellaneous
Systemic diseases
  Endocrine disorders
    Addison's disease
    Hyperthyroidism
    Hypoparathyroidism
  Collagen-vascular disorders
    Systemic lupus erythematosus
    Scleroderma
    Polyarteritis nodosa
  Others
    Acquired immunodeficiency syndrome (AIDS)
    Uremia
    Neuropathic disorders (especially diabetes mellitus,
        amyloidosis, postvagotomy state)
    Cirrhosis
    Chronic cholecystitis
    Deficiency syndromes
      Pernicious anemia
      Pellagra
    Immunoglobulin deficiencies
Drugs (see also Acute Diarrhea above)
  Chronic opiate abuse
Collagenous colitis
Eosinophilic gastroenteritis
Protein-losing enteropathy

References
1. Fine KD, Krejs GJ, Fordtran JS: In general reference 12,
   p 290.
2. Donowitz M: Pathophysiology of Diarrhea. In general reference 13, p 73.

6-G. Maldigestion, Malabsorption Syndromes

Maldigestion Syndromes
Pancreatic disorders
  Chronic pancreatitis
  Pancreatic resection
  Pancreatic carcinoma
  Cystic fibrosis
  Nonbeta islet cell tumors
  Severe protein malnutrition
  Effect of vagotomy on pancreatic secretion
Hepatobiliary disease
  Extrahepatic biliary obstruction
  Chronic intrahepatic cholestasis (e.g., primary biliary cirrhosis)
  Severe hepatocellular injury
Impaired enzyme or bile salt function due to:
  Inadequate mixing (e.g., following gastrectomy, gastrojejunostomy, vagotomy, pyloroplasty, Billroth I or II)
  Acid pH in small bowel (e.g., Zollinger-Ellison syndrome)
  Ileal resection
  Severe diffuse ileal disease (e.g., Crohn's disease)

Malabsorption Syndromes
Mucosal cell abnormality
  Sprue
    Celiac
    Tropical
    Collagenous
  Whipple's disease
  Inflammatory diseases
    Crohn's disease
    Infectious enteritis
      Bacterial
      Mycobacterial
      Parasitic (e.g., *Giardia, Cryptosporidia*)
      Viral (e.g., cytomegalovirus [CMV])
Short-bowel syndrome
  Massive resection (especially for Crohn's disease)
  Enteroenteric fistulas
  Jejunoileal bypass surgery
  Gastroileal anastomosis (inadvertent)
Bacterial overgrowth as a result of stasis
  Surgical blind loop
  Stricture, fistula
  Crohn's disease

        Small-bowel diverticula
        Hypomotility states
            Intestinal diabetic neuropathy
            Scleroderma
            Intestinal pseudoobstruction
    Disaccharidase deficiency
        Lactase
        Sucrase-isomaltase
    Others
        Ischemic bowel disease
        Radiation enteritis
        Nongranulomatous ulcerative jejunitis
        Abetalipoproteinemia
        Hypogammaglobulinemia
        Chloridorrhea, congenital or acquired
        HIV-related
Infiltrative diseases
    Lymphoma
        Primary intestinal
        Extraintestinal
    Amyloidosis
    Eosinophilic gastroenteritis
    Mastocytosis
Intestinal congestion
    Congestive heart failure
    Constrictive pericarditis
Lymphatic obstruction
    Intestinal lymphangiectasia
    Tuberculosis
    Retroperitoneal malignancy

Systemic Disorders
Endocrine disorders
    Diabetes mellitus
    Hypoparathyroidism
    Hyperthyroidism
    Hypothyroidism
    Adrenal insufficiency
Protein malnutrition
Collagen-vascular disease
    Systemic lupus erythematosus
    Scleroderma
    Polyarteritis nodosa
    Rheumatoid arthritis
    Vasculitis
Dermatologic disorders
    Dermatitis herpetiformis
    Psoriasis

Food allergy
Others
   Pernicious anemia
   Carcinoid syndrome
   Iron deficiency
   Dysgammaglobulinemia, heavy-chain
   Genetic disorders of membrane transport (e.g., Hartnup
     disease)

Drugs
Cholestyramine
Colchicine
Broad-spectrum antibiotics (e.g., neomycin)
Cytotoxic drugs
Irritant laxatives
Phenindione
Methotrexate
Mefenamic acid
Alcohol

References
1. Wright TL, Heyworth MF: Maldigestion and Malabsorption. In general reference 12, p 263.
2. Symposium on Malabsorption. *Am J Med* 67:979, 1979.
3. Eastwood GL: Malabsorption Syndrome. In general reference 13, p 89.

6-H. Gastrointestinal Bleeding

Upper Gastrointestinal Bleeding
Acute (these account for > 90% of cases)
- Peptic ulcer disease
- Erosive gastritis
- Ruptured esophagogastric varices
- Mallory-Weiss tear
- Erosive esophagitis

Chronic/occult sources
- Peptic ulcer disease
  - Esophagitis/esophageal ulcer
  - Duodenitis/duodenal ulcer
  - Gastritis/gastric ulcer
  - Stress ulceration
  - Marginal/stomal ulceration
  - Intestinal ulceration (e.g., associated with use of enteric-coated potassium chloride and nonsteroidal antiinflammatory drugs [NSAIDs])
- Erosive gastritis, duodenitis
  - Peptic
  - Alcohol
  - Drug-induced
    - Acetylsalicylic acid
    - NSAIDs
- Esophageal sources
  - Gastroesophageal reflux
  - Barrett's esophagitis
  - Candidal esophagitis
  - Herpetic esophagitis
  - Esophageal rupture (Boerhaave syndrome)
  - Graft-versus-host disease
- Neoplasms
  - Carcinoma of esophagus, stomach, small intestine
  - Polyps (primarily gastric)
  - Leiomyoma
  - Lymphoma
  - Sarcoma
  - Neurofibroma
  - Carcinoid
  - Hemangioma
  - Plasmacytoma
  - Infiltrative extraintestinal neoplasms
- Ischemic bowel disease (especially mesenteric vascular occlusion)

Bleeding disorders (e.g., anticoagulant therapy)
Others
    Aortointestinal fistula
      Leaking aneurysm
      Aortic prosthesis
    Osler-Rendu-Weber syndrome
    Hereditary telangiectasis
    Angiodysplasia
    Uremia
    Amyloidosis
    Hemobilia
      Traumatic
      Ruptured hepatic artery aneurysm
    Vasculitis (especially polyarteritis nodosa, systemic
      lupus erythematosus)
    Blue rubber nevus bleb syndrome
    Esophagogastric varices after partial sclerotherapy
    Epistaxis with swallowed blood
    Ehlers-Danlos syndrome
    Pseudoxanthoma elasticum
    Hemoptysis
    Intramural hematomas
    Whipple's disease

Lower Gastrointestinal Bleeding

Acute (these account for > 90% of cases)
    Diverticulosis
    Ischemic colitis
    Angiodysplasia
    Colonic polyps
    Carcinoma
    Hemorrhoids
    Radiation colitis
Chronic/occult sources
    Anorectal lesions
      Hemorrhoids
      Anal fissures/fistulas
      Proctitis
      Trauma
      Rectal carcinoid tumor
      Solitary rectal ulcer syndrome
    Colonic lesions
      Neoplasms
        Carcinoma of rectum, colon
        Polyps
          Tubular adenomas
          Villous adenomas

   Familial colonic polyposis
   Gardner's syndrome
   Peutz-Jeghers syndrome
   Juvenile polyposis
  Others
   Leiomyoma
   Sarcoma
   Lymphoma
   Neurofibroma
   Hemangioma
 Chronic inflammatory bowel disease
  Ulcerative colitis
  Crohn's disease
 Infectious colitis
  Bacterial (especially *Shigella*, *Salmonella*, pathogenic *Escherichia coli*)
  Mycobacterial (especially tuberculosis)
  Parasitic (especially amebiasis, schistosomiasis, whipworm)
  Spirochetal (especially syphilis)
  Viral (cytomegalovirus, herpes simplex virus)
 Ischemic colitis (e.g., mesenteric artery occlusion)
 Pseudomembranous colitis
 Radiation colitis
Diverticular disease
 Diverticulitis
 Meckel's diverticulum
Mechanical abnormalities
 Incarcerated hernia
 Volvulus
 Intussusception
 Foreign body
Systemic diseases
 Bleeding disorder (see 8-O)
 Uremia
 Amyloidosis
 Vasculitis
  Polyarteritis nodosa
  Systemic lupus erythematosus
  Henoch-Schönlein purpura
  Dermatomyositis
Others
 Aortointestinal fistula
 Arteriovenous malformation
 Osler-Rendu-Weber syndrome
 Submucosal vascular ectasia (angiodysplasia)
 Blue rubber nevus bleb syndrome

Pseudoxanthoma elasticum
Ehlers-Danlos syndrome
Whipple's disease

References
1. Peterson WL: Gastrointestinal Bleeding. In general reference 12, p 397.
2. Eastwood GL: Gastrointestinal Bleeding. In general reference 13, p 216.

6-I. Abdominal Distention

Mechanical Bowel Obstruction
Extraluminal compression
  Adhesions
    Postsurgical
    Inflammatory
    Neoplastic
    Congenital
  Intraabdominal abscess
  Hematoma
  Neoplasm
  Pregnancy
  Annular pancreas
  Superior mesenteric artery (SMA) syndrome
Intraluminal obstruction
  Neoplasm
    Benign
    Malignant
  Inflammatory disorders (e.g., Crohn's disease, ulcerative colitis, diverticulitis)
  Trauma
  Foreign body
  Gallstones
  Parasites (especially *Ascaris*)
  Fecaliths
  Enteroliths
  Bezoars
  Food boluses
  Meconium
  Pneumatosis intestinalis
Intussusception
Volvulus
Hernias
Obstruction at surgical anastomosis

Congenital defect (e.g., Hirschsprung's disease)
Others
　Radiation stenosis
　Endometriosis

Adynamic Ileus, Nonmechanical Obstruction
Intraabdominal causes
　Peritoneal inflammation (see 6-J)
　Traumatic
　　Postoperative
　　Penetrating wounds
　Bacterial infections
　Chemical irritants
　　Blood
　　Gastric contents (perforated ulcer)
　　Bile
　　Pancreatic enzymes (acute pancreatitis)
　Vascular insufficiency
　　Strangulation
　　　Intramural (distention resulting from mechanical
　　　　ileus)
　　　Extramural (compression of mesenteric vessels)
　　Mesenteric artery thrombosis or embolus
　Retroperitoneal irritation
　　Retroperitoneal hemorrhage
　　Psoas abscess
　　Pyelonephritis
　　Renal colic
　　Perinephric abscess
　　Pancreatitis
　　Pancreatic abscess
　　Cancer
　　Lymphoma
Extraabdominal causes
　Mechnical ventilation
　Toxic, metabolic
　　Pneumonia
　　Empyema
　　Uremia
　　Porphyria
　　Severe systemic infection
　　Heavy metal poisoning (e.g., lead)
　Traumatic
　　Thoracic
　　Retroperitoneal
　　Intracranial
　　Spinal
　Severe electrolyte imbalance (e.g., hypokalemia)

Other
  Osteomyelitis of spine

Vascular Obstruction
Mesenteric artery thrombosis or embolus
Venous thrombosis

Idiopathic Intestinal Pseudoobstruction

Excessive Intraluminal Gas
Aerophagia
Increased intestinal gas production

Ascites (see 6-Q)

Reference
1. Jones RS, Schirmer BD: Intestinal Obstruction, Pseudoobstruction, and Ileus. In general reference 12, p 369.

6-J. Peritonitis

Infections
  Bacterial
    Acute bacterial peritonitis
    Spontaneous bacterial peritonitis (SBP), usually in cir-
      rhotics with ascites
    Secondary bacterial peritonitis (associated with perfo-
      ration)
  Mycobacterial (primarily tuberculosis)
  Fungal (rare), especially:
    Candidiasis
    Histoplasmosis
    Cryptococcosis
    Coccidioidomycosis
  Parasitic (rare), especially:
    Schistosomiasis
    Ascariasis
    Enterobiasis
    Amebiasis
    Strongyloidiasis
Spontaneous perforation of viscus
  Peptic ulcer disease
  Appendicitis
  Gangrenous cholecystitis
  Diverticulitis

Strangulated bowel
  Small-bowel adhesion
  Incarcerated hernia
  Volvulus
Perforating carcinoma
Ulcerative colitis (especially with toxic megacolon)
Ischemic bowel
Ingested foreign body
Meckel's diverticulum
Ruptured visceral abscess or cyst, especially:
  Liver
  Kidney
  Spleen
  Tuboovarian
Trauma, iatrogenic
  Penetrating wounds
  Surgical injury, including laparoscopic surgery
  Instrumentation
    Sigmoidoscopy or colonoscopy
    Gastroscopy
    Abortion
    Paracentesis
Neoplasms
  Primary mesothelioma
  Secondary carcinomatosis
  Pseudomyxoma peritonei
Vasculitis
  Systemic lupus erythematosus
  Allergic vasculitis (Henoch-Schönlein purpura)
  Köhlmeier-Degos disease
Granulomatous peritonitis
  Parasitic infestations
  Sarcoidosis
  Tumors
  Crohn's disease
  Starch granules
Gynecologic disorders
  Endometriosis
  Teratoma
  Leiomyomatosis
  Dermoid cyst
  Melanosis
Chemical irritants
  Bile
  Blood
  Gastric juice
  Barium
  Enema or douche contents

Others
  Chronic peritoneal dialysis
  Eosinophilic peritonitis
  Chylous peritonitis (see 6-Q, under Chylous ascites)
  Whipple's disease
  Sclerosing peritonitis
  Peritoneal lymphangiectasis
  Peritoneal encapsulation
  Peritoneal loose bodies and peritoneal cysts
  Mesothelial hyperplasia and metaplasia
  Splenosis
  Familial paroxysmal polyserositis (familial Mediterranean
      fever)

Reference
1. Bender MD: Diseases of the Peritoneum, Mesentery and
   Diaphragm. In general reference 12, p 1932.

6-K. Pancreatitis

Biliary tract disease
  Gallstone pancreatitis
  Choledocholithiasis
Alcoholic pancreatitis
  Acute
  Chronic recurrent (relapsing)
Idiopathic
Peptic ulcer disease (especially penetrating duodenal or
      gastric ulcer)
Trauma
  Blunt or penetrating
  Surgical
Duodenal disease
  Sphincter of Oddi dysfunction
  Sphincter of Oddi obstruction
    Fibrosis, stenosis
    Edema
    Tumor
  Crohn's disease
  Periampullary diverticulum
Neoplasm
  Head of pancreas
  Pancreatic carcinoma with duct obstruction

Carcinoma of ampulla of Vater
  Metastatic carcinoma
Congenital pancreatic disorders
  Pancreas divisum
  Hereditary (familial) pancreatitis
Acquired pancreatic disorders
  Fibrosis
  Calculi
  Ductal strictures
  Pseudocyst
  Abscess
Metabolic disorders
  Hyperlipoproteinemia (types I, IV, and V)
  Hyperparathyroidism
  Other hypercalcemic states
Drugs
  Azathioprine
  Thiazide diuretics
  Ethacrynic acid
  Furosemide
  Tetracycline
  Salicylazosulfapyridine
  L-Asparaginase
  Oral contraceptives
  Corticosteroids
  Estrogens
Toxins
  Methyl alcohol
  Scorpion venom (Trinidad)
Infectious agents
  Mumps
  Coxsackie B infection
  Viral hepatitis
  Legionnaire's disease
  Campylobacter
  Mycoplasma
  Ascaris infestation
Vascular insufficiency or infarction
Miscellaneous
  Protein-calorie malnutrition
  Pregnancy
  Hypothermia
  Cardiopulmonary bypass surgery
  Hypotensive shock
  Endoscopic retrograde cholangiopancreatography
  Upper gastrointestinal endoscopy
  Posttransplantation
  AIDS

References
1. Salt WB, Schenker S: Amylase—Its Clinical Significance: A Review of the Literature. *Medicine* 55:269, 1976.
2. The Pancreas. In general reference 12, p 1765.
3. Steinberg WM: Acute Pancreatitis. In general reference 13, p 233.

6-L. Hyperamylasemia Not Associated with Pancreatitis

Intraabdominal Disorders
Biliary tract disease, common duct stones
Perforated peptic ulcer not in contact with pancreas
Intestinal infarction
Intestinal obstruction
Intestinal perforation
Afferent loop syndrome
Ruptured ectopic pregnancy
Salpingitis
Dissecting aortic aneurysm
Peritonitis
Appendicitis

Salivary Gland Disorders
Parotitis (especially mumps)
Calculi
Radiation sialoadenitis
Maxillofacial surgery
Drugs
   Oxyphenbutazone
   Phenylbutazone

Miscellaneous
Chronic renal insufficiency
Salivary-type hyperamylasemia
Malignancy (especially lung)
Macroamylasemia
Cerebral trauma
Burns
Traumatic shock
Postoperative hyperamylasemia
Diabetic ketoacidosis
Renal transplantation

Pneumonia
Acquired bisalbuminemia
Prostatic disease
Pregnancy
Drugs
    Opiates

Reference
1. Salt WB, Schenker S: Amylase—Its Clinical Significance:
    A Review of the Literature. *Medicine* 55:269, 1976.

6-M. Hepatomegaly

Palpable Liver Without Hepatic Pathology
Normal variant
Thin or flaccid abdominal wall
Depressed right diaphragm (e.g., emphysema)
Subdiaphragmatic lesion (e.g., abscess)
Riedel's lobe

True Hepatic Enlargement
Inflammatory liver disease
    Hepatitis (see 6-O)
        Infectious
            Viral
            Schistosomiasis
            Other
        Alcoholic
        Other toxins
        Drug-induced
        Autoimmune
        Other
    Abscess
        Pyogenic
        Amebic
    Cholangitis
        Suppurative
        Sclerosing
    Pericholangitis (especially ulcerative colitis)
Chronic liver disease, cirrhosis (see 6-P)
    Alcoholic
    Posthepatitic
    Postnecrotic
    Cholestatic

    Metabolic disorders
    Other causes
Extrahepatic biliary obstruction
    Choledocholithiasis
    Biliary stricture
    Pancreatitis
    Carcinoma
        Bile ducts
        Head of pancreas
        Ampulla of Vater
    External compression
Hepatic congestion
    Congestive heart failure
    Constrictive pericarditis
    Budd-Chiari syndrome (hepatic outflow obstruction)
        Thrombosis
        Tumor
    Venoocclusive disease
Infiltrative disorders, storage diseases
    Lipid accumulation
        Fatty liver
            Alcohol
            Diabetes mellitus
            Obesity
            Severe protein malnutrition
            Nonalcoholic steatonecrosis
            Jejunoileal bypass
            Parenteral hyperalimentation
            Corticosteroids, Cushing's syndrome
            Fatty liver of pregnancy
            Massive tetracycline therapy
            Toxins (e.g., carbon tetrachloride, DDT)
            Reye's syndrome
        Lipid storage disease (especially Gaucher's disease, Niemann-Pick disease)
    Glycogen accumulation
        Glycogen storage disease
        Diabetic glycogenosis
    Granulomatous infiltration (especially sarcoidosis, miliary tuberculosis, disseminated fungal diseases, some drug reactions)
    Myelo- and lymphoproliferative disorders
        Lymphoma
        Myeloid metaplasia
        Multiple myeloma
        Leukemia
    Amyloidosis
    Congenital hepatic fibrosis

    Hemochromatosis
    Wilson's disease
    Alpha$_1$-antitrypsin deficiency
    Hurler's syndrome
Neoplasms
    Primary
        Malignant
            Hepatocellular carcinoma
            Cholangiocarcinoma
            Angiosarcoma
        Benign
            Adenoma
            Hemangioma
            Focal nodular hyperplasia
    Metastatic
        Pancreas
        Colon
        Lung
        Breast
        Stomach
        Kidney
        Esophagus
        Carcinoid
Cysts
    Congenital
        Solitary
        Polycystic
    Acquired (especially echinococcal)

References

1. Isselbacher KJ: Jaundice and Hepatomegaly. In general reference 1, p 264.
2. General reference 14.

6-N. Jaundice

Primarily Unconjugated Hyperbilirubinemia
Increased production
  Hemolysis, intravascular or extravascular (see 8-B)
  Ineffective erythropoiesis
  Hematomas, pulmonary embolus
Decreased hepatic uptake
  Gilbert's syndrome
  Drugs
    Flavaspidic acid
    Iodinated contrast agents
    Rifampin
  Decreased cystolic binding proteins (e.g., newborn or
      premature infants)
  Portocaval shunt
  Prolonged fasting
Decreased glucuronidation
  Crigler-Najjar syndrome, types I and II
  Gilbert's syndrome
  Physiologic jaundice of newborn
  Breast-milk jaundice
  Hepatic parenchymal disease
  Noncirrhotic portal fibrosis

Primarily Conjugated Hyperbilirubinemia
Decreased liver excretion, intrahepatic
  Familial or hereditary disorders
    Dubin-Johnson syndrome
    Rotor syndrome
    Benign recurrent intrahepatic cholestasis
    Intrahepatic cholestasis of pregnancy
  Acquired disorders
    Hepatitis (see 6-O)
    Cirrhosis (see 6-P)
    Alcoholic liver disease
    Primary sclerosing cholangitis
    Pericholangitis
    Drugs and toxins, especially:
      Chlorpromazine
      Erythromycin estolate
      Isoniazid
      Halothane
  Others
    Hepatic malignancy, primary or metastatic

Congestive heart failure
Shock
Sepsis
Toxemia of pregnancy
Hepatic trauma
Sarcoidosis
Amyloidosis
Sickle cell hepatopathy
Postoperative jaundice
Total parenteral nutrition
Idiopathic cholestasis associated with lymphoma
Intrahepatic biliary obstruction
    Primary biliary cirrhosis
    Primary sclerosing cholangitis
    Liver allograft rejection
    Graft-versus-host disease
    Ductopenic syndromes (e.g., Alagille's syndrome)
    Neoplasms (primary, metastatic, lymphoma)
Extrahepatic biliary obstruction
  Congenital
    Biliary atresia
    Idiopathic dilatation of common bile duct
    Cystic fibrosis
    Choledochal cysts
  Acquired
    Cholecystitis
    Common bile duct obstruction
      Choledocholithiasis
      Tumors (benign, malignant)
        Gallbladder
        Bile ducts
        Ampulla of Vater
        Pancreas
        Lymphoma
        Metastatic tumors
      External compression
      Strictures
        Common bile duct
        Sphincter of Oddi
        Primary sclerosing cholangitis
        AIDS (*Cryptosporidium*)
      Pancreatitis
      Parasites (*Ascaris*)

References

1. Walkoff AW (ed): Bilirubin Metabolism and Hyperbilirubinemia. *Semin Liver Dis,* Vol 3, No 1, 1983.

2. General reference 14.
3. Zawacki JK: Jaundice and Bilirubin Metabolism. In general reference 13, p 281.

6-O. Hepatitis, Abnormal "Liver Function Tests"

Causes of Acute Liver Injury with ALT or AST > 1000 μ/L
Acute viral hepatitis
Ischemic hepatopathy ("shock" liver)
Toxin, drug-induced
Autoimmune hepatitis (occasional)
Choledocholithiasis (initial, rare)

Causes of Chronic Active Hepatitis
Viral (type B or C)
Drug-induced
Wilson's disease
Alpha₁-antitrypsin deficiency
Autoimmune hepatitis

Infection
Viral
   Hepatitis A
   Hepatitis B
   Hepatitis C
   Hepatitis D (delta, only with HB$_s$Ag)
   Hepatitis E (underdeveloped countries)
   Infectious mononucleosis (Epstein-Barr virus)
   Cytomegalovirus
   Varicella zoster
   Coxsackie
   Rubella
   Measles
   Herpes simplex
   Other
Bacterial (not necessarily hepatitis, per se)
   Pyogenic abscesses
      Numerous aerobic and anaerobic organisms

Hepatic dysfunction in bacterial sepsis
  Escherichia coli
  Klebsiella pneumoniae
  Pseudomonas aeruginosa
  Proteus species
  Bacteroides species
  Staphylococcus aureus
  Aerobic and anaerobic streptococci
Hepatic dysfunction in gram-positive infections
  Pneumococcal
  Streptococcal
  Staphylococcal
  Clostridia species
Hepatic dysfunction in gram-negative infections
  E. coli
  Paracolon bacteria
  P. aeruginosa
  Proteus
  Bacteroides
  Aerobacter
  Klebsiella
  Enterobacteriaceae
  Salmonella
  Gonococcal
  Legionnaires' bacillus
  Other
    Brucellosis
    Typhoid fever
    Tularemia
Mycobacterial
  Tuberculosis
  Leprosy
Spirochetal
  Syphilis (congenital, secondary, or late)
  Leptospirosis
  Relapsing fever (*Borrelia* species)
Mycotic
  Histoplasmosis
  Coccidioidomycosis
  Blastomycosis
  Nocardiosis
  Cryptococcosis
  Candidiasis
  Actinomycosis
Parasitic (e.g., malaria, toxoplasmosis, amebiasis, schisto-
    somiasis, others)
Rickettsial (e.g., Q fever)

Toxins
Industrial toxins (e.g., carbon tetrachloride, yellow phosphorus, trichloroethylene)
Plant toxins
  Mushrooms (e.g., *Amanita phalloides*)
  Aflatoxin

Drug-induced Liver Disease, Including Hepatitis
Drugs implicated in the etiology of chronic liver injury
  Acetaminophen
  Aspirin
  Dantrolene
  Ethanol
  Isoniazid
  Methyldopa
  Nitrofurantoin
  Oxyphenisatin
  Perhexiline maleate
  Propylthiouracil
  Sulfonamides
Specific classes of drugs associated with acute and/or
      chronic liver dysfunction
  Anesthetics
    Chloroform
    Halothane
    Enflurane
    Methoxyflurane
    Cyclopropane
  Analgesics, antiinflammatory agents
    Acetaminophen
    Salicylates
    Propoxyphene
    Phenylbutazone
    Indomethacin
    Ibuprofen
    Naproxen
    Sulindac
  Antibacterial agents
    Erythromycin
      Estolate
      Ethylsuccinate
      Lactobionate
    Tetracyclines
    Nitrofurantoins
    Sulfonamides
    Penicillin

Oxacillin
Cloxacillin
Carbenicillin
Chloramphenicol
Clindamycin
Antituberculous agents
Isoniazid
Rifampin
Ethionamide
Paraaminosalicylic acid
Pyrazinamide
Antifungal, antiparasitic agents
Antimony
Arsenic
Thiobendazole
Hycanthone
5-Fluorocytosine
Quinacrine
Griseofulvin
Ketoconazole
Anticonvulsants
Phenytoin
Valproic acid
Trimethadione
Antihypertensives, diuretics
Chlorothiazide
Furosemide
Chlorthalidone
Methyldopa
Hydralazine
Captopril
Antiarrhythmic agents
Quinidine
Aprindine
Procainamide
Amiodarone
Antimetabolites
6-Mercaptopurine
Methotrexate
Azathioprine
6-Thioguanine
Chlorambucil
5-Fluorouracil
Nitrogen mustard
Cyclophosphamide
Hormones
Androgens (e.g., methyltestosterone)

Corticosteroids
Estrogens
Oral hypoglycemics
  Chlorpropamide
  Tolbutamide
  Tolazamide
  Acetohexamide
  Glyburide
Antithyroid drugs
  Methimazole
  Carbimazole
  Propylthiouracil
Psychoactive agents
  Phenothiazines (especially chlorpromazine)
  Imipramine
  Benzodiazepines
  Meprobamate
  Monoamine oxidase inhibitors
  Haloperidol
  Diazepam
  Chlordiazepoxide
  Desipramine
  Amitriptyline
Others
  Doxapram
  Cimetidine
  Ranitidine
  Perhexiline maleate
  Cinchophen
  Gold salts
  Allopurinol
  Pyridium
  Papaverine
  Oxyphenisatin
  Nicotinic acid
  Disulfiram

Others
Autoimmune hepatitis
Wilson's disease
Granulomatous hepatitis of unknown etiology
Hepatitis associated with systemic disorders
  Hyperthermia
  Cardiac failure
  Shock
  Burns

Hyperthyroidism
Hypoxia

References
1. Gitlin N: Clinical Aspects of Liver Disease Caused by Industrial and Environmental Toxins. In general reference 14, p 791.
2. Bass NM, Ockner RK: Drug-induced Liver Disease. In general reference 14, p 754.
3. Koff RS: Viral Hepatitis. In general reference 13, p 326.
4. Patwardhan RV, Tomaiolo PP: Alcohol and Drug-Induced Liver Disease. In general reference 13, p 356.

6-P. Cirrhosis, Chronic Liver Disease

Alcoholic
Infectious
   Viral hepatitis (especially B and C)
   Schistosomiasis
   Other infections (uncommon; e.g., congenital syphilis, brucellosis)
Biliary
   Primary biliary cirrhosis
   Primary sclerosing cholangitis
   Secondary biliary cirrhosis (chronic extrahepatic obstruction)
Autoimmune chronic active hepatitis
"Cryptogenic" cirrhosis
   Posthepatitic (non-B, non-C)
   Postnecrotic
Chemical
   Toxins
      Alcohol
      Carbon tetrachloride
      Dimethylnitrosamine
      Phosphorus
      Vinyl chloride
      Arsenic

Beryllium
Pesticides
Drugs
  Halothane
  Isoniazid
  Methotrexate
  Methyldopa
  Monamine oxidase inhibitors
  Nitrofurantoin
  Oxyphenisatin
Congestive
  Severe chronic right heart failure
    Tricuspid insufficiency
    Constrictive pericarditis
    Cor pulmonale
    Mitral stenosis
  Hepatic vein obstruction (Budd-Chiari syndrome)
  Venooclusive disease
Hereditary or familial disorders
  Hepatolenticular degeneration (Wilson's disease)
  Cystic fibrosis
  Alpha$_1$-antitrypsin deficiency
  Hemochromatosis
  Galactosemia
  Glycogen storage diseases
  Hereditary fructose intolerance
  Tyrosinosis
  Hypervitaminosis A
  Thalassemia (secondary iron overload)
  Sickle cell disease
  Osler-Rendu-Weber syndrome
  Abetalipoproteinemia
Others
  Sarcoidosis
  Granulomatous cirrhosis
  Congenital hepatic fibrosis
  Indian childhood cirrhosis
  Nutritional (e.g., jejunoileal bypass surgery)
  Nonalcoholic steatohepatitis

References
1. Galambos JT: Cirrhosis. In Smith LH (ed): *Major Problems in Internal Medicine.* Philadelphia: Saunders, 1979, vol. 17.
2. General reference 14.

3. Tomaiolo PP, Patwardhan RV: Consequences of Chronic Liver Disease. In general reference 13, p 384.

6-Q. Ascites

Without Peritoneal Disease
Portal hypertension
  Cirrhosis (see 6-P)
  Alcoholic hepatitis
  Hepatic congestion
    Congestive heart failure
    Tricuspid insufficiency
    Constrictive pericarditis
    Inferior vena cava obstruction
    Hepatic vein obstruction (Budd-Chiari syndrome)
    Cardiomyopathy
  Portal vein occlusion
    Thrombosis
    Tumor
  Idiopathic tropical splenomegaly
  Partial nodular transformation
  Hypervitaminosis A
  Fulminant hepatic failure
  Idiopathic
Hypoalbuminemia
  Cirrhosis (see 6-P)
  Nephrotic syndrome
  Protein-losing enteropathy
  Lymphangiectasia
  Severe malnutrition
Miscellaneous
  Myxedema
  Hepatocellular carcinoma (usually with cirrhosis)
  Ovarian disease
    Tumor (Meigs' syndrome)
    Struma ovarii
    Ovarian overstimulation syndrome
  Pancreatic ascites
    Rupture of pseudocyst
    Leak from pancreatic duct

Bile ascites
  Gallbladder rupture
  Traumatic bile leak
Chylous ascites
  Rupture (traumatic, surgical) of abdominal lymphatics
  Congenital lymphangiectasia
  Obstructed lymphatics (especially secondary to malignancy, tuberculosis, filariasis)
  Constrictive pericarditis
  Cirrhosis
  Sarcoidosis

With Peritoneal Disease
Infection
  Mycobacterial
  Bacterial
    Primary (spontaneous bacterial peritonitis [SBP] in cirrhosis)
    Secondary (ruptured viscus)
  Fungal (rare, especially candidiasis, histoplasmosis, cryptococcosis)
  Parasitic (rare, especially schistosomiasis, ascariasis, enterobiasis)
  AIDS
Neoplasm
  Primary mesothelioma
  Metastatic carcinomatosis
    Ovarian
    Pancreatic
    Gastric
    Colonic
    Lymphoma
Miscellaneous
  Peritoneal vasculitides
    Systemic lupus erythematosus
    Henoch-Schönlein purpura
    Köhlmeier-Degos disease
  Eosinophilic peritonitis
  Familial Mediterranean fever
  Pseudomyxoma peritonei
  Whipple's disease
  Granulomatous peritonitis
    Foreign bodies (especially starch)
    Sarcoidosis

Gynecologic lesions (especially endometriosis, ruptured
    dermoid cyst)
Peritoneal lymphangiectasis

References

1. Bender MD: Diseases of the Peritoneum, Mesentery, and
Diaphragm. In general reference 12, p 1932.
2. General reference 14.

6-R. Ascitic Fluid Characteristics in Various Disease States[a]

Condition	Gross appearance	Protein (gm/dl)[b]	Cell count		Other
			RBCs (> 10,000/mm³)	WBCs	
Hepatic cirrhosis	Straw-colored or bile-stained	< 2.5 (95%)[a]	1%	< 250/mm³ (90%)[a]; predominantly mononuclear	pH gradient < 0.1[c]
Congestive heart failure	Straw-colored	Variable, 1.5–5.3	10%	< 1000/mm³ (90%); usually mesothelial, mononuclear	
Nephrogenic ascites	Straw-colored or chylous[d]	< 2.5 (100%)	Unusual	< 250/mm³; mesothelial, mononuclear	
Neoplasm	Straw-colored, hemorrhagic, mucinous, or chylous[d]	> 2.5 (75%)	20%	> 1000/mm³ (50%); variable cell types	Cytology, cell block, peritoneal biopsy

Peritonitis, bacterial	Turbid or purulent	If purulent, > 2.5	Unusual	> 500/mm³ with > 250 neutrophils/mm³	Gram's stain, culture; pH gradient > 0.1[c]
Peritonitis, tuberculous	Clear, turbid, hemorrhagic, or chylous[d]	> 2.5 (50%)	7%	> 1000/mm³ (70%); usually > 70% lymphocytes	Peritoneal biopsy, stain and culture for acid-fast bacilli
Pancreatic ascites	Turbid, hemorrhagic, or chylous[d]	Variable, often > 2.5	Variable, may be blood-stained	Variable	↑↑ amylase in ascitic fluid, ↑ in serum

↑ = increased; ↑↑ = greatly increased.

[a]Because the conditions of examining and selecting patients were not identical in each series, the percentage figures (in parentheses) should be taken as an indication of the order of magnitude rather than as the precise incidence of any abnormal finding.

[b]Ascit ic fluid is generally classified as transudative if the protein content < 2.5 gm/dl and the serum-fluid albumin gradient > 1.1 gm/dl, and as exudative if protein > 2.5 gm/dl and serum-fluid albumin gradient < 1.1 gm/dl. Transudates are usually found in cirrhosis, in congestive heart failure, and with nephrogenic ascites; exudates, in neoplastic states and with peritonitis and pancreatic ascites.

[c]pH gradient = blood pH − ascitic fluid pH.

[d]If ascitic fluid is chylous (milky in appearance), then triglyceride content determination and lipoprotein electrophoresis should be performed.

Source: Modified from Glickman RM, Isselbacher KJ: Abdominal Swelling and Ascites. In Wilson JD, et al (eds): Harrison's Principles of Internal Medicine (12th ed). New York: McGraw-Hill, 1991, p 269. Copyright © 1991 by McGraw-Hill Book Co.

7 GENITOURINARY SYSTEM

7-A. Hematuria

Pseudohematuria (Dyes and Pigments)
Beets
Food dyes
Phenolphthalein
Rifampin
Pyridium
Urates
Porphyrins
Myoglobin
Free hemoglobin (intravascular hemolysis)

Renal Parenchymal Causes
Primary glomerulopathy
   Postinfectious glomerulonephritis
   Benign recurrent hematuria
   Berger's disease (IgA nephropathy)
   Membranoproliferative glomerulonephritis
   Focal glomerulosclerosis
   Crescentic glomerulonephritis
Multisystem and hereditary diseases
   Diabetes mellitus
   Lupus erythematosus

    Goodpasture's syndrome
    Polyarteritis nodosa, other vasculitides
    Endocarditis, shunt nephritis
    Hemolytic-uremic syndrome
    Henoch-Schönlein purpura
    Malignant hypertension
    Polycystic kidney disease
    Hereditary nephritis (Alport's syndrome)
    Fabry's disease
    Nail-patella syndrome
Other
    Exercise
    Pyelonephritis, acute
    Nephrolithiasis
    Renal cyst
    Renal trauma
    Renal neoplasm
    Coagulopathy, thrombocytopenia
    Interstitial nephritis, acute
    Analgesic nephropathy
    Sickle cell trait or disease
    Medullary sponge kidney
    Lymphomatous or leukemic infiltration
    Hydronephrosis
    Oxaluria
    Vascular anomalies, intrarenal arteriovenous fistula
    Acute febrile illnesses (especially malaria, yellow fever, smallpox)
    Papillary necrosis
    Renal infarction (acute renal artery occlusion, renal vein thrombosis)
    Renal transplant rejection

Lower Urinary Tract Causes

Congenital anomalies (e.g., ureterocele)
Neoplasms (bladder, ureter, prostate, urethral), benign or malignant
Cystitis, prostatitis, urethritis
Calculi
Trauma
Foreign body
Coagulopathy
Varices (renal pelvis, ureter, bladder)
Radiation cystitis
Drugs (especially cyclophosphamide, anticoagulants)
Schistosomiasis
Genitourinary tuberculosis

Non–Urinary Tract Causes
Neoplasm of adjacent organs
Diverticulitis
Pelvic inflammatory disease
Appendicitis

Reference
1. Glassock RJ, et al: Primary Glomerular Diseases. In general reference 15, p 1182.

7-B. Polyuria

Central diabetes insipidus (see 4-H)
Renal disease
   Nephrogenic diabetes insipidus, congenital
   Chronic renal insufficiency (especially tubulointerstitial disease)
   Diuretic phase of acute renal failure
   Postobstructive diuresis, partial or intermittent obstruction
   Hypercalcemic nephropathy
   Hypokalemic nephropathy
   Sickle cell trait or disease
   Multiple myeloma
   Amyloidosis
   Sarcoidosis
   Sjögren's syndrome
   Decreased protein intake
Osmotic diuresis
   Diabetes mellitus, poorly controlled
   Mannitol or urea administration
   Iodinated contrast dye
   Hyperalimentation
   Tube feedings
Drugs
   Alcohol
   Diuretics
   Lithium
   Demeclocycline
   Methicillin
   Gentamicin
   Amphotericin B
   Phenothiazines
   Sulfonylurea compounds

Phenytoin
Propoxyphene
Methoxyflurane
Colchicine
Vinblastine
Clonidine
Norepinephrine
Narcotic antagonists
Water load
  Psychogenic polydipsia
  Intravenous fluid therapy
  Drug-induced polydipsia (e.g., phenothiazines, anticho-
    linergics)
  Resorption of edema fluid

Reference

1. Berl T, Schrier RW: Disorders of Water Metabolism. In
   general reference 16, p 1.

7-C. Proteinuria

Benign/Physiologic
Fever
Exercise
Orthostatic
Contrast dye

Usually Nonnephrotic
Chronic pyelonephritis
Other interstitial nephritis (acute or chronic)
Arteriolar nephrosclerosis
Malignant hypertension
Interstitial nephritis
Acute tubular necrosis
Urinary tract obstruction
Nephrolithiasis
Renal neoplasm
Renal trauma
Polycystic kidney disease
Hereditary nephritis (Alport's syndrome)
Glomerular disease, especially:
  IgA nephropathy (Berger's disease)
  Crescentic glomerulonephritis

Hemolytic-uremic syndrome
Scleroderma
Genitourinary tuberculosis

Often Nephrotic

Primary renal disease, especially:
  Minimal change disease
  Membranous glomerulopathy
  Membranoproliferative glomerulonephritis
  Focal glomerulosclerosis
Systemic disease, especially:
  Diabetes mellitus
  Lupus erythematosus
  Polyarteritis nodosa
  Wegener's granulomatosis
  Henoch-Schönlein purpura
  Mixed cryoglobulinemia
  Amyloidosis (primary or secondary)
  Neoplasm
    Solid tumors (especially lung, colon, stomach, breast)
    Hodgkin's disease, other lymphomas
    Multiple myeloma
  Sarcoidosis
  Myxedema
  Graves' disease
  Sickle cell disease
Toxins, drugs
  Gold
  Mercury
  Heroin
  Nonsteroidal antiinflammatory drugs
  Tolbutamide, chlorpropamide
  Rifampin
  Probenecid
  Penicillamine
  Captopril
  Trimethadione and other anticonvulsants
  Lithium
Allergens
  Pollens
  Poison ivy and oak
  Snake venom
  Bee or insect stings
  Antitoxin (e.g., tetanus toxoid)
Infection, especially:
  Bacterial (e.g., streptococcal, staphylococcal)
  Hepatitis B

    Cytomegalovirus
    Epstein-Barr virus (infectious mononucleosis)
    Human immunodeficiency virus (HIV)
    Syphilis
    Malaria
    Helminthic (e.g., schistosomiasis)
    Leprosy
Miscellaneous
    Congestive heart failure
    Tricuspid insufficiency
    Constrictive pericarditis
    Preeclampsia
    Renal vein thrombosis, inferior vena cava obstruction
    Massive obesity
    Hereditary diseases, especially:
       Congenital nephrotic syndrome
       Alport's syndrome
       Fabry's disease
       Alpha$_1$-antitrypsin deficiency
       Nail-patella syndrome

Reference

1. Glassock RJ, et al: Primary Glomerular Diseases. In general reference 15, p 1182.

7-D. Glomerulopathy

Primary Renal Disease

Minimal change disease
Membranous glomerulopathy
Membranoproliferative glomerulonephritis
Focal glomerulosclerosis
Crescentic glomerulonephritis
Mesangial proliferative glomerulonephritis (e.g., IgA nephropathy)

Infection

Bacterial, especially:
    Streptococcal
    Endocarditis
    Shunt infection
    Septicemia, especially pneumococcal or staphylococcal
    Meningitis
Viral, especially:
    Hepatitis

Mononucleosis
Rubella
Varicella
Mumps
Cytomegalovirus
HIV infection
Syphilis
Parasitic infestation (especially malaria)
Tuberculosis

Systemic Disease
Diabetes mellitus
Lupus erythematosus
Scleroderma
Rheumatoid arthritis
Mixed connective tissue disease
Polyarteritis nodosa
Wegener's granulomatosis
Hemolytic-uremic syndrome
Thrombotic thrombocytopenic purpura
Henoch-Schönlein purpura
Mixed cryoglobulinemia
Goodpasture's syndrome
Waldenström's macroglobulinemia
Amyloidosis
Neoplasm
    Solid tumors (especially lung, stomach, colon, breast)
    Hodgkin's disease, other lymphoma
    Multiple myeloma, light chain nephropathy
Sarcoidosis
Preeclampsia
Postpartum renal failure
Sickle cell disease
Hepatic cirrhosis

Drugs, Toxins
Mercury
Gold
Penicillamine
Probenecid
Heroin
Amphetamines
Trimethadione
Sulfonamides

Other
Radiation
Hereditary nephritis (Alport's syndrome)

Fabry's disease
Nail-patella syndrome
Congenital nephrotic syndrome
Renal transplant rejection

References
1. Glassock RJ, et al: Primary Glomerular Diseases. In
   general reference 15, p 1182.
2. Glassock RJ, et al: Secondary Glomerular Diseases. In
   general reference 15, p 1280.

7-E. Interstitial Nephropathy

Infection
    Bacterial (pyelonephritis, acute or chronic)
    Mycoplasmal
    Toxoplasmosis
    Leptospirosis
    Brucellosis
    Mononucleosis
    Legionnaires' disease
Urinary tract obstruction, vesicoureteral reflux
Papillary necrosis
Drugs
    Analgesics (especially aspirin, phenacetin)
    Methicillin and penicillin analogues
    Cephalosporins
    Tetracycline
    Rifampin
    Amphotericin B
    Furosemide
    Thiazides
    Nonsteroidal antiinflammatory agents
    Allopurinol
    Phenytoin
    Azathioprine
    Lithium
    Phenindione
    Warfarin
    Paraaminosalicylic acid
    Polymyxins
Heavy metals
    Lead
    Cadmium
    Uranium

Copper
Beryllium
Oxalate deposition
  Hereditary
  Small-bowel disease or resection
  Ethylene glycol intoxication
  Methoxyflurane anesthesia
Uric acid deposition
  Gout
  Chemotherapy of leukemia or lymphoma
Hypercalcemia
  Hyperparathyroidism
  Neoplasm, multiple myeloma
  Milk-alkali syndrome
  Sarcoidosis
Hypokalemia
Radiation
Neoplastic disease
  Multiple myeloma
  Light chain nephropathy
  Leukemic or lymphomatous infiltration
  Waldenström's macroglobulinemia
Vascular causes
  Arteriolar nephrosclerosis
  Renal artery stenosis
  Atheroembolic disease
  Sickle cell trait or disease
Hereditary causes
  Hereditary nephritis
  Medullary sponge kidney
  Medullary cystic disease
  Polycystic kidney disease
  Cystinosis
  Fabry's disease
Systemic lupus erythematosus
Mixed cryoglobulinemia
Sarcoidosis
Sjögren's syndrome
Amyloidosis
Balkan nephropathy
Transplant rejection

Reference

1. Bennett WM, Elzinga LW, Porter GA: Tubulointerstitial
   Disease and Toxic Nephropathy. In general reference 15,
   p 1430.

7-F. Renal Tubular Acidosis

Distal (Type I)
Pyelonephritis, chronic
Obstructive uropathy
Drugs, toxins
  Amphotericin B
  Analgesics
  Toluene
  Lithium
  Cyclamate
Nephrocalcinosis, especially:
  Primary hyperparathyroidism
  Vitamin D intoxication
  Primary hypercalciuria
  Medullary sponge kidney
  Hyperthyroidism
Autoimmune diseases
  Hypergammaglobulinemic states, especially:
    Hyperglobulinemic purpura
    Cryoglobulinemia
    Familial hypergammaglobulinemia
  Systemic lupus erythematosus
  Sjögren's syndrome
  Thyroiditis
  Chronic active hepatitis
  Primary biliary cirrhosis
  Diffuse interstitial pulmonary fibrosis
Genetically transmitted diseases
  Sickle cell disease
  Ehlers-Danlos syndrome
  Hereditary elliptocytosis
  Fabry's disease
  Wilson's disease
  Medullary cystic disease
  Hereditary fructose intolerance
Hepatic cirrhosis
Balkan nephropathy
Oxalate nephropathy
Multiple myeloma
Renal transplantation
Idiopathic (sporadic or hereditary)

Proximal (Type II)
Primary (sporadic or hereditary)
Transient (infants)

Carbonic anhydrase deficiency (e.g., genetic or acetazol-
    amide-induced)
Fanconi syndrome (multiple proximal tubular defects)
    Drugs and toxins
        Outdated tetracycline
        Toluene
        Gentamicin
        Streptozotocin
        Lead
        Cadmium
        Mercury
    Multiple myeloma
    Amyloidosis
    Sjögren's syndrome
    Vitamin D–deficient, –dependent, and –resistant states
    Cystinosis
    Tyrosinemia
    Lowe's syndrome
    Wilson's disease
    Hereditary fructose intolerance
    Pyruvate carboxylase deficiency
    Medullary cystic disease
    Paroxysmal nocturnal hemoglobinuria
    Osteopetrosis
    Renal transplantation

Type IV
Aldosterone deficiency
    Adrenal insufficiency
    Adrenal enzyme deficiency, congenital adrenal hyperpla-
        sia, especially 21-hydroxylase deficiency
    Selective aldosterone deficiency
        Hyporeninemic hypoaldosteronism
            Diabetes
            Tubulointerstitial disease
            Nonsteroidal antiinflammatory drugs
            Cyclosporine
            HIV infection
            Sickle cell disease
            Obstructive uropathy
        Heparin
        ACE inhibitors
Mineralocorticoid resistance
    Pseudohypoaldosteronism
    Obstructive uropathy
    Sickle cell disease
    Drugs (spironolactone, triamterene, amiloride)

References
1. Cogan MG, Rector FC: Acid-Base Disorders. In general reference 15, p 737.
2. Shapiro JI, Kaehny WD: Pathogenesis and Management of Metabolic Acidosis and Alkalosis. In general reference 16, p 161.
3. Rose BD: *Clinical Physiology of Acid-Base and Electrolyte Disorders* (3rd ed). New York: McGraw-Hill, 1989, p 501.

7-G. Urinary Tract Obstruction

Urethral
Congenital urethral stenosis, web, atresia
Posterior urethral valves
Inflammation or stricture
Trauma

Bladder Neck
Prostatic hypertrophy, prostatitis
Carcinoma (prostate, bladder)
Bladder infection
Functional
  Neuropathy (peripheral neuropathy, spinal cord injury or
    trauma)
  Drugs (parasympatholytics, ganglionic blockers)

Ureteral
Ureteral-pelvic junction stricture
Intraureteral
  Clots
  Stones
  Crystals (e.g., sulfa, uric acid)
  Papillae (necrosed)
  Trauma (edema, stricture)
  Tumor
  Foreign bodies
Extraureteral
  Endometriosis
  Retroperitoneal tumor or metastases, especially:
    Cervical
    Endometrial
    Ovarian
    Prostatic

Lymphoma
Sarcoma
Fibrosis
Idiopathic
Associated with inflammation, drugs (e.g., methyser-
gide), radiation, inflammatory bowel disease
Pregnancy
Aortic or iliac aneurysm
Surgical ligation
Retroperitoneal hemorrhage

References

1. Brenner BM, Milford EL, Seifter JL: Urinary Tract Obstruction. In general reference 1, p 1206.
2. Klahr S: Obstructive Nephropathy: Pathophysiology and
Management. In general reference 16, p 581.

7-H. Nephrolithiasis

Calcium-Containing Stones

Idiopathic
Primary hypercalciuria (absorptive, renal-leak) with or with-
out hyperuricosuria
Hypercalcemic states (see 1-L)
Primary hyperparathyroidism
Malignancy
Immobilization
Milk-alkali syndrome
Vitamin D excess
Sarcoidosis
Hyperthyroidism
Renal tubular acidosis, distal
Medullary sponge kidney
Carbonic anhydrase inhibitors (e.g., acetazolamide)
Cushing's disease or syndrome
Hypoparathyroidism
Hyperoxaluria
Primary (congenital)
Increased metabolic production (e.g., ethylene glycol or
methoxyflurane excess)
Increased gastrointestinal absorption
Increased dietary intake
Small-bowel disease or resection (e.g., jejunoileal by-
pass, celiac sprue, regional enteritis)

Calcium-Magnesium-Ammonium Phosphate Stones (Struvite)
Chronic infection (usually with urea-splitting organisms, e.g., *Proteus, Klebsiella, Pseudomonas*), especially associated with:
  Chronic Foley catheter use
  Ileal loop

Uric Acid and/or Xanthine Stones
Gout
Leukemia, lymphoma (especially after chemotherapy)
Purine pathway enzyme deficiency states
  Lesch-Nyhan syndrome
  Glycogen storage disease
  Xanthinuria
Drugs (e.g., aspirin, probenecid)
Gastrointestinal disorders associated with chronic diarrhea (especially with ileostomy)

Cystine Stones
Cystinuria

Reference
1. Pac CYC: Urolithiasis. In Schrier RW, Gottschalk CW (eds): *Diseases of the Kidney* (5th ed). Boston: Little, Brown, 1993, p 729.

7-I. Acute Renal Failure

Prerenal Azotemia
Hypovolemia
   Hemorrhage
   Gastrointestinal losses
   Sweating
   Diuretic use
   Third-spacing (e.g., intestinal ileus)
   Burns
Decreased effective circulating volume
   Cirrhosis/ascites, hepatorenal syndrome
   Nephrotic syndrome
   Cardiac causes (e.g., congestive heart failure, acute
     myocardial infarction, pericardial tamponade)
Catabolic states, e.g.:
   Starvation with stress
   Sepsis, serious infection
   Postsurgical state
   Steroids
   Tetracycline
Breakdown of blood in gastrointestinal tract or resorption of
   hematoma

Drugs, Toxins
Heavy metals
   Mercury
   Arsenic
   Lead
   Cadmium
   Uranium
   Bismuth
   Copper
   Platinum
Carbon tetrachloride, other organic solvents
Ethylene glycol
Pesticides
Fungicides
X-ray contrast media (iodinated)
Antibiotics
   Penicillin
   Tetracycline
   Aminoglycosides
   Cephalosporins
   Amphotericin B
   Sulfonamides

Rifampin
Polymyxin
Other drugs
Nonsteroidal antiinflammatory agents
Captopril
Phenytoin
Phenindione
Methoxyflurane
Furosemide
EDTA

Ischemic Disorders
Major trauma, surgery
Massive hemorrhage, severe volume depletion
Pancreatitis
Septic shock
Crush injury
Hemolysis, transfusion reaction
Rhabdomyolysis

Glomerular/Vascular Diseases
Poststreptococcal glomerulonephritis
Systemic lupus erythematosus
Scleroderma
Polyarteritis nodosa, hypersensitivity angiitis
Henoch-Schönlein purpura
Bacterial endocarditis
Serum sickness
Goodpasture's syndrome
Crescentic glomerulonephritis, idiopathic
Wegener's granulomatosis
Drug-induced vasculitis
Malignant hypertension
Hemolytic-uremic syndrome
Thrombotic thrombocytopenic purpura
Preeclampsia
Abruptio placentae
Postpartum renal failure
Transplant rejection

Interstitial/Intratubular Diseases
Interstitial nephritis (see 7-E), especially:
Infection
Drugs
Oxalate deposition
Hypercalcemia
Multiple myeloma

Pyelonephritis, papillary necrosis
Hyperuricemia
Radiation

Major Vessel Diseases
Renal artery thrombi, emboli, stenosis
Renal vein or inferior vena cava thrombosis
Dissecting aneurysm (aorta with or without renal arteries)

Postrenal Causes*
Urethral obstruction
Bladder neck obstruction
Ureteral obstruction

References
1. Brezis M, Rosen S, Epstein FH: Acute Renal Failure. In general reference 15, p 993.
2. Conger JD, Briner VA, Schrier RW: Acute Renal Failure: Pathogenesis, Diagnosis, and Management. In general reference 16, p 495.

*See 7-G.

7-J. Renal Failure, Reversible Factors

Infection, upper or lower urinary tract
Obstruction
Volume depletion
Drugs, toxins
Congestive heart failure
Hypertension
Pericardial tamponade
Hypercalcemia
Hyperuricemia ($> 15-20$ mg/dl)
Hypokalemia

Reference
1. Alfrey AC, Chan L: Chronic Renal Failure: Manifestations and Pathogenesis. In general reference 16, p 539.

7-K. Urinary Diagnostic Indices[a]

	Prerenal azotemia	Oliguric acute renal failure
Urine osmolality (mOsm/kg H_2O)	> 500	< 350
Urine Na^+ (mEq/L)	< 20	> 40
Urine/plasma urea nitrogen	> 8	< 3
Urine/plasma creatinine	> 40	< 20
Fractional excretion of Na^+ (%)[b]	< 1	> 1

[a]These indices are useful only in oliguric states.
[b]Fractional excretion of Na^+ =

$$\frac{(\text{urine } Na^+ \text{ concentration}) (\text{plasma creatinine concentration})}{(\text{plasma } Na^+ \text{ concentration}) (\text{urine creatinine concentration})} \times 100\%.$$

Source: Modified from Miller TR, et al: Urinary Diagnostic Indices in Acute Renal Failure: A Prospective Study. *Ann Intern Med* 89:49, 1978.

7-L. Chronic Renal Failure

Glomerulopathy, primary renal*
Glomerulopathy associated with systemic disease*
Genetically transmitted disease
  Polycystic kidney disease
  Hereditary nephritis
  Fabry's disease
  Oxalosis
  Cystinosis
  Medullary cystic disease
  Medullary sponge kidney
  Nail-patella syndrome
  Congenital nephrotic syndrome
Vascular diseases
  Nephrosclerosis
  Malignant hypertension
  Cortical necrosis
  Renal artery stenosis, thrombosis, emboli
  Renal vein thrombosis, inferior vena cava thrombosis

Interstitial disease†
   Drugs: analgesics, lithium, amphotericin B
   Heavy metals: lead, cadmium, beryllium
Urinary tract obstruction‡

References
1. General reference 15.
2. General reference 16.

*See 7-D.
†See 7-E.
‡See 7-G.

7-M. Indications for Dialysis

Biochemical Criteria
Volume overload
Serum K^+ > 6 mEq/L (despite medical management)
Serum HCO_3^- < 10 mEq/L, pH < 7.20
Blood urea nitrogen > 100–200 mg/dl
Serum creatinine > 10–20 mg/dl

Symptomatic Criteria
Central nervous system symptoms (e.g., lethargy, confusion, seizures, asterixis)
Gastrointestinal symptoms (e.g., nausea, vomiting)
Pericarditis
Bleeding diathesis

Miscellaneous Indications (Conditions Not Necessarily Associated with Renal Failure)
Hypercalcemia
Hypermagnesemia
Hyperuricemia
Hypernatremia
Hypothermia
Drug overdose, toxin ingestion

Reference
1. Shinaborger JH: Indications for Dialysis. In Massry SG, Sellers AL (eds): *Clinical Aspects of Uremia and Dialysis.* Springfield, Ill.: Thomas, 1976, p 490.

7-N. Impotence

Aging
Psychogenic causes
Testicular causes (primary or secondary)
    Congenital hypogonadism (especially Froehlich's syndrome, Klinefelter's syndrome, hypogonadotropic eunuchoidism)
    Acquired hypogonadism
      Viral orchitis
      Trauma
      Radiation
      Hepatic insufficiency
      Chronic pulmonary disease
      Chronic renal failure
      Granulomatous disease (especially leprosy)
    Testicular carcinoma
    Pituitary tumor, especially when associated with hyperprolactinemia
    Pituitary insufficiency
Neurologic disease
    Anterior temporal lobe lesion
    Spinal cord disease (e.g., multiple sclerosis)
    Loss of sensory input
      Diabetes mellitus
      Polyneuropathy
      Tabes dorsalis
      Dorsal root ganglia disease
    Lesions of nervi erigentes
      Aortic bypass surgery
      Total prostatectomy
      Rectosigmoid surgery
Drugs
    Estrogens
      Anticholinergic agents
      Antidepressants (e.g., amitriptyline, doxepin)
      Antihypertensive agents
        Guanethidine
        Methyldopa
        Clonidine
        Reserpine
        Propranolol
        Thiazides
        Spironolactone
      Antipsychotic agents (e.g., phenothiazines, haloperidol, thioridazine)

Tranquilizers (e.g., diazepam, chlordiazepoxide, barbiturates)
Addictive drugs (e.g., heroin, methadone)
Alcoholism
Vascular disease (e.g., Leriche syndrome)
Priapism, previous
Penile disease
  Trauma
  Peyronie's disease

Reference
1. McConnell JD, Wilson JD: Impotence and Infertility in Men. In general reference 1, p 296.

7-O. Menorrhagia and Nonmenstrual Vaginal Bleeding

Ovulatory Bleeding
Midcycle ovulatory bleeding (normal variant)
Inadequate corpus luteum (luteal phase defect)
Uterine or endometrial disease
  Endometritis
  Endometriosis
  Uterine adenomyosis
  Endometrial polyps
  Uterine leiomyomas
  Carcinoma
  Intrauterine synechiae
  Intrauterine device
Vaginal or cervical disease
  Vaginitis, cervicitis
  Cervical scarring
  Carcinoma

Anovulatory
Estrogen withdrawal bleeding
Estrogen breakthrough bleeding
  Chronic, continuous estrogen therapy
  Polycystic ovarian disease
  Estrogen-secreting ovarian tumor
Progesterone breakthrough bleeding (e.g., continuous low-dose oral contraceptives)
Abortion
Ectopic pregnancy

Ovarian destructive lesions (e.g., tumor, chronic salpingo-oophoritis)

Hypothalamic or pituitary lesion (e.g., tumor, sarcoidosis)

Adrenal disease (hyper- or hypofunction)

Thyroid disease (hyper- or hypofunction)

Stress, psychogenic factors

References

1. Carr BR, Wilson JD: Disorders of the Ovary and Female Reproductive Tract. In general reference 1, p 1776.
2. Riddick DH: Disorders of Menstrual Function. In Danforth DN, Scott JR (eds): *Obstetrics and Gynecology* (5th ed). Philadelphia: Lippincott, 1986, p 873.

8 HEMATOLOGIC SYSTEM

8-A. Anemia—Hypoproliferative (Low Reticulocyte Count)

Nutrient Deficiency
Iron deficiency
  Chronic blood loss
  Pregnancy
  Dietary deficiency
  Malabsorption
    Subtotal gastrectomy
    Malabsorption syndromes
  Hemoglobinuria/hemosiderinuria
    Intravascular hemolysis
  Hemodialysis
Vitamin B_{12} deficiency
  Dietary deficiency (rare)
  Impaired absorption
    Insufficient intrinsic factor
      Pernicious anemia
      Gastrectomy (total or partial)
      Gastric mucosal injury (e.g., lye ingestion)
      Congenital
    Malabsorption syndromes
      Sprue, tropical or nontropical

        Ileal resection
        Regional ileitis
        Infiltrative intestinal disease (e.g., lymphoma)
        Chronic pancreatitis
        Familial selective malabsorption
        Drug-induced malabsorption
      Competitive absorption
        Diphyllobothrium latum (fish tapeworm)
        Blind-loop syndromes
    Increased requirements
      Pregnancy
      Neoplasia
Folate deficiency
    Dietary deficiency (especially in alcoholics, infants)
    Impaired absorption
      Malabsorption syndromes
        Sprue, tropical or nontropical
        Whipple's disease
        Small-intestinal resection
        Infiltrative intestinal disease (e.g., lymphoma)
        Scleroderma
        Amyloidosis
      Drug-induced malabsorption (anticonvulsants)
    Increased requirements
      Pregnancy
      Infancy
      Hemolytic anemia
      Chronic exfoliative dermatitis
      Neoplasia
      Uremia
    Impaired metabolism
      Trimethoprim
      Methotrexate
      Pyrimethamine
      Alcohol
Other nutritional deficiencies
    Vitamin A
    Pyridoxine (rare)
    Vitamin C
    Starvation
    Protein deficiency (kwashiorkor)

Anemia of Chronic Disease

Chronic infection
    Subacute bacterial endocarditis
    Osteomyelitis
    Chronic pyelonephritis
    Chronic pulmonary infection

Tuberculosis
Chronic fungal infection
Pelvic inflammatory disease
Chronic inflammatory diseases
Rheumatoid arthritis
Rheumatic fever
Systemic lupus erythematosus
Vasculitis
Inflammatory bowel disease
Acquired immunodeficiency syndrome (AIDS)/HIV infection
Malignancy
Chronic renal disease
Chronic liver disease
Endocrine dysfunction
Hypothyroidism
Adrenal insufficiency
Panhypopituitarism
Hyperparathyroidism

Bone Marrow Disorders
Congenital
Red cell aplasia (Diamond-Blackfan anemia)
Congenital dyserythropoietic anemias
Hereditary sideroblastic anemias
Aplastic
Pancytopenia (see 8-L)
Pure red cell aplasia
Congenital (Diamond-Blackfan anemia)
Acquired
Associated with thymoma, chronic lymphocytic leukemia, etc.
Drug-induced
Toxic
Megaloblastic
Antimetabolites (e.g., 5-fluorouracil, 6-thioguanine, 6-mercaptopurine, azathioprine)
Sideroblastic (e.g., alcohol, lead, isoniazid, chloramphenicol)
Aplastic (see 8-L)
Infiltrative, with or without fibrosis
Infection
Tuberculosis
Fungal disease
Gaucher's and other lipid storage diseases
Malignancy
Hematologic (leukemia, lymphoma, myeloma)
Marrow metastases

Neoplastic
  Leukemia, acute and chronic
  Lymphoproliferative disorders
    Lymphoma, with marrow involvement
      Hodgkin's disease
      Non-Hodgkin's lymphoma
    Plasma cell myeloma
    Hairy-cell leukemia
  Myeloproliferative disorders
    Agnogenic myeloid metaplasia with fibrosis
    Essential thrombocythemia
    Chronic myelogenous leukemia
  Myelodysplastic syndromes
    Refractory anemia (RA)
    RA with ringed sideroblasts
    RA with excess of blasts (RAEB)
    RAEB in transformation
    Chronic myelomonocytic leukemia

Other
Marathon runner's anemia (physiologic)

References
1. Aboulafia DM, Mitsuyasu RT: Hematologic Abnormalities in AIDS. *Hematol Oncol Clin N Am* 5:195, 1991.
2. Erslev AJ: Anemia of Chronic Renal Failure; Anemia of Endocrine Disorders; Anemia of Chronic Disorders. In general reference 18, pp 438, 444, 540.
3. Fairbanks VF, Beutler E: Iron Deficiency. In general reference 18, p 482.
4. Lee GR: The Anemia of Chronic Disorders. In general reference 17, p 840.
5. Herbert V: Hematologic Complications of Alcoholism I, II. *Semin Hematol,* vol. 17, 1980.
6. Dressendorfer RH, Wade CE, Amsterdam EA: Development of Pseudoanemia in Marathon Runners During a 20-day Road Race. *JAMA* 246:1215, 1981.
7. Jandl JH (ed): *Blood: Textbook of Hematology.* Boston: Little, Brown, 1987.

8-B. Anemia—Hyperproliferative (Increased Reticulocyte Count)

Blood Loss

Hypersplenism

Hemolytic Anemia
Hereditary
  Membrane abnormalities
    Hereditary spherocytosis
    Hereditary elliptocytosis
    Hereditary stomatocytosis
    Acanthocytosis (abetalipoproteinemia)
    Others
  Enzyme deficiencies
    Glucose-6-phosphate dehydrogenase
    Pyruvate kinase
    Others
  Hemoglobinopathies
    Qualitative
      Sickle-cell anemia
      Hemoglobin C disease
      Unstable hemoglobin disease
      Others
    Unbalanced chain synthesis
      Thalassemias
Acquired
  Nonimmune
    Traumatic
      Prosthetic valves and other cardiac abnormalities
      March hemoglobinuria
      Burns
    Microangiopathic hemolytic anemia
      Disseminated intravascular coagulation
      Thrombotic thrombocytopenic purpura
      Hemolytic uremic syndrome
      Vasculitis
      Malignant hypertension
    Infectious agents
      Malaria
      Clostridium perfringens
      Bartonella
      Babesiosis
      Others
    Chemical agents
      Naphthalene

    Arsine
    Copper
    Chlorates
    Venoms
    Distilled water (IV)
    Others
  Paroxysmal nocturnal hemoglobinuria
  Hypophosphatemia
  "Spur cell" anemia (liver disease)
Immune
  Warm antibody mediated
    Incompatible blood transfusion
    Hemolytic disease of newborn
    Idiopathic
    Secondary
      Infectious
        Viral (e.g., Epstein-Barr virus, cytomegalovirus)
      Collagen-vascular disorders
        Systemic lupus erythematosus
        Rheumatoid arthritis
      Malignancy
        Lymphoproliferative disorders
        Solid tumors
      Other
        Sarcoidosis
        Inflammatory bowel disease
      Drugs (many)
  Cold antibody mediated
    Idiopathic
    Secondary
      Infectious
        Viral (e.g., Epstein-Barr virus)
        Mycoplasma pneumoniae
      Malignancy
    Paroxysmal cold hemoglobinuria

References

1. Lee GR: Introduction to the Hemolytic Anemias. In general reference 17, p 944.
2. Beutler E: Glucose-6-phosphate Dehydrogenase Deficiency. In general reference 18, p 591.
3. Packman CH, Leddy JP: Acquired Hemolytic Anemia due to Warm-reacting Autoantibodies; Cryopathic Hemolytic Syndromes; Drug-related Immunologic Injury of Erythrocytes. In general reference 18, pp 666, 675, 681.

8-C. Polycythemia

Spurious
   Decreased plasma volume (e.g., dehydration, burns)
   "Stress" erythrocytosis (Gaisböck's syndrome)
Secondary
   Appropriate (associated with tissue hypoxia)
      Decreased arterial PO_2
         Altitude
         Chronic pulmonary disease
         Alveolar hypoventilation
         Cyanotic congenital heart disease
      Normal arterial PO_2
         Carboxyhemoglobinemia (e.g., cigarette smoking)
         Hemoglobinopathies (with an increased affinity for
            oxygen)
         Cobalt ingestion
   Inappropriate
      Renal disorders
         Hydronephrosis
         Renal cysts
         Renal cell carcinoma
      Endocrine disorders
         Cushing's syndrome
         Primary hyperaldosteronism
         Pheochromocytoma
         Androgen therapy
      Hepatoma
      Cerebellar hemangioblastoma
      Uterine leiomyoma
      Familial erythrocytosis
Primary
   Polycythemia rubra vera

References

1. Athens JW, Lee GR: Polycythemia: Erythrocytosis. In general reference 17, p 1245.
2. Erslev AJ: Erythrocyte Disorders—Erythrocytosis. In general reference 18, p 705.

8-D. Granulocytopenia

Infections
  Viral
    Influenza
    Infectious mononucleosis
    Infectious hepatitis
    Rubella
    Chickenpox
    Smallpox
    Poliomyelitis
    Others
  Bacterial
    Overwhelming bacteremia
    Typhoid fever
    Tularemia
    Brucellosis
  Mycobacterial
    Miliary tuberculosis
  Rickettsial
  Protozoan
    Malaria
Chemical agents, drugs, physical agents
  Predictable
    Antineoplastic agents
    Benzene
    Ionizing radiation
  Idiosyncratic
    Aminopyrine
    Phenothiazines
    Antithyroid drugs
    Sulfonamides
    Anticonvulsants
    Antibiotics
    Ethanol
    Others
Systemic illness
  Systemic lupus erythematosus
  Felty's syndrome
  AIDS/HIV infection
Hypersplenism
Nutritional
  B_{12} or folate deficiency
  Cachexia
  Alcoholism
Bone marrow dysfunction
  Acute leukemias (aleukemic)

Lymphoproliferative disorders
Myelofibrosis
  Primary—myeloproliferative disorders
  Secondary
    Tumor infiltration
    Infection
Aplastic anemia
Myelodysplastic syndromes
Immune neutropenia
  Drug-induced
  Collagen vascular disease (systemic lupus erythemato-
    sus)
  Neoplasia
  Autoimmune neutropenia
Other
  Benign neutropenia of blacks
  Chronic idiopathic neutropenia
  Cyclic neutropenia
  Benign familial neutropenia

References

1. Dale DC: Neutropenia. In general reference 18, p 807.
2. Budman DR, Steinberg AD: Hematologic Aspects of Systemic Lupus Erythematosus. *Ann Intern Med* 86:220, 1977.
3. Aboulafia DM, Mitsuyasu RT: Hematologic Abnormalities in AIDS. *Hematol Oncol Clin N Am* 5:195, 1991.

8-E. Granulocytosis

Reactive
Infection
  Bacterial (primarily)
  Mycobacterial
  Fungal
  Rickettsial
  Viral
  Spirochetal
  Parasitic
Physical stimuli
  Exercise
  Trauma
  Seizures
Inflammation, acute and chronic
  Collagen vascular disorders
  Hypersensitivity reactions
  Gout
  Vasculitis
  Nephritis
  Inflammatory bowel disease
  Hepatitis
  Pancreatitis
  Dermatitis
Neoplasm
Tissue necrosis
  Myocardial infarction
  Gangrene
  Burns
Drugs, toxins, especially:
  Corticosteroids
  Epinephrine
  Lithium
  Endotoxin
  Histamine
  Lead
  Growth factors (granulocyte colony-stimulating factor
    [G-CSF], granulocyte-macrophage colony-stimulating
    factor [GM-CSF])
Hematologic disorders
  Hemorrhage
  Postsplenectomy, functional asplenia
  Recovery from agranulocytosis
  Hemolytic anemia
  Bone marrow infiltration (e.g., solid tumor, tuberculosis)

Metabolic disorders
  Diabetic ketoacidosis
  Cushing's syndrome
  Eclampsia
  Uremia
  Thyroid storm
Pregnancy

Autonomous
Myeloproliferative disorders
  Chronic myelogenous leukemia
  Polycythemia rubra vera
  Agnogenic myeloid metaplasia
  Essential thrombocythemia
Acute leukemia

Congenital Causes

Reference
1. Dale DC: Neutrophilia. In general reference 18, p 816.

8-F. Lymphocytosis

Infections
  Viral
    Infectious mononucleosis
    Infectious lymphocytosis
    Cytomegalovirus infection
    Mumps
    Measles
    Chickenpox
    Viral hepatitis
    Others
  Bacterial
    Pertussis
    Brucellosis
    Tuberculosis
  Spirochetal
    Syphilis, secondary and congenital
  Protozoan
    Toxoplasmosis
Hematologic disorders
  Lymphocytic leukemia, acute and chronic
  Non-Hodgkin's lymphoma with marrow involvement

Drug hypersensitivity
  Phenytoin
  p-Aminosalicylic acid
Miscellaneous
  Thyrotoxicosis
  Post–cardiopulmonary bypass syndrome
  Serum sickness
  Immune thrombocytopenic purpura
  Immune hemolytic anemia

Reference

1. Williams WJ: Lymphocytosis. In general reference 18, p 963.

8-G. Lymphocytopenia

Immunodeficiency syndromes
  AIDS/HIV infection
  Congenital immunodeficiency syndromes
    Wiskott-Aldrich syndrome
    Ataxia-telangiectasia
    DiGeorge's syndrome
  Common variable immunodeficiency
Increased lymphocyte destruction
  Radiation therapy
  Antineoplastic chemotherapy
  Antilymphocyte/antithymocyte globulin
  Corticosteroid or adrenocorticotropic hormone adminis-
    tration or excess
Increased lymphocyte loss
  Thoracic duct drainage
  Intestinal lymphectasia
  Intestinal lymphatic obstruction (e.g., lymphoma)
  Whipple's disease
  Severe right-sided heart failure
    Tricuspid insufficiency
    Constrictive pericarditis
Other
  Sarcoidosis
  Advanced malignancy
  Miliary tuberculosis
  Renal failure
  Aplastic anemia
  Collagen-vascular disorders
    Systemic lupus erythematosus

References
1. Williams WJ: Lymphocytopenia. In general reference 18, p 964.
2. Spivak JL, Bender BS, Quinn TC: Hematologic Abnormalities in the Acquired Immune Deficiency Syndrome. *Am J Med* 77:224, 1984.

8-H. Monocytosis

Infections
   Tuberculosis
   Subacute bacterial endocarditis
   Syphilis
Hematologic disorders
   Myelodysplastic syndromes
   Acute nonlymphocytic leukemia (especially acute monocytic leukemia)
   Myeloproliferative disorders
   Lymphoproliferative disorders
      Hodgkin's disease
      Non-Hodgkin's lymphoma
      Myeloma
   Malignant histiocytosis
   Postsplenectomy
   Recovery from neutropenia
      Infectious
      Drug-induced
      Postchemotherapy
      Growth factor use (GM-CSF)
   Benign familial neutropenia
Collagen-vascular disorders
   Rheumatoid arthritis
   Systemic lupus erythematosus
   Temporal arteritis
   Polyarteritis nodosa
   Polymyositis
Malignancy
   Any solid tumor
Gastrointestinal disorders
   Sprue
   Ulcerative colitis
   Regional enteritis
Miscellaneous
   Sarcoidosis

Reference
1. Lichtman MA: Monocytosis and Monocytopenia. In general reference 18, p 882.

8-I. Eosinophilia

Infections
  Bacterial
    Scarlet fever
    Tuberculosis
    Leprosy
    Others
  Parasitic
    Protozoans (e.g., toxoplasmosis, amebiasis, malaria)
    Metazoans (e.g., trichinosis, filariasis, schistosomiasis)
    Arthropods (e.g., scabies)
Allergic disorders
  Hay fever
  Asthma
  Bronchopulmonary aspergillosis
  Urticaria
  Angioneurotic edema
  Serum sickness
  Food allergy
Skin disorders
  Psoriasis
  Eczema
  Erythema multiforme
  Dermatitis herpetiformis
  Exfoliative dermatitis
  Pityriasis rosea
  Ichthyosis
  Pemphigus vulgaris
  Facial granuloma
Drug reactions
Hematologic disorders
  Myeloproliferative disorders
  Lymphoproliferative disorders
  Acute nonlymphocytic leukemia
  Myelodysplastic syndromes
  Postsplenectomy
  Hypereosinophilic syndrome
Malignancy
  Advanced solid tumors

Collagen-vascular disorders
  Rheumatoid arthritis
  Polyarteritis nodosa
  Vasculitis
  Dermatomyositis
  Systemic lupus erythematosus
  Eosinophilic fasciitis
Gastrointestinal disorders
  Eosinophilic gastroenteritis
  Ulcerative colitis
  Regional enteritis
Others
  Adrenal insufficiency
  Loeffler's syndrome
  Chronic eosinophilic pneumonia
  Sarcoidosis
  Radiation therapy
  Chronic renal disease
  Familial eosinophilia
  Eosinophilia-myalgia syndrome

References

1. Zucker-Franklin D: Eosinopenia and Eosinophilia. In general reference 18, p 845.
2. Chusid MJ, et al: The Hypereosinophilic Syndrome. *Medicine* 54:1, 1975.
3. Pearson DJ, Rosenow EC: Chronic Eosinophilic Pneumonia (Carrington's): A Follow-up Study. *Mayo Clin Proc* 53:73, 1978.

8-J. Thrombocytopenia

Decreased Production
Primary hematologic disorders
  Aplastic anemia
  Acute leukemia
  Lymphoproliferative disorders
    Lymphoma
    Myeloma
    Chronic lymphocytic leukemia
  Myeloproliferative disorders
    Agnogenic myeloid metaplasia with myelofibrosis
    Chronic myelogenous leukemia (accelerated phase)
  Myelodysplastic syndromes
  Selective megakaryocytic aplasia
Bone marrow infiltration
  Solid tumor
  Infection
    Tuberculosis
    Other
  Gaucher's disease
  Osteopetrosis
Drugs
  Selective megakaryocytic suppression
    Thiazides
    Alcohol
    Estrogens
    Interferon
  Nonselective myelosuppression
    Predictable (e.g., antineoplastic chemotherapy)
    Idiosyncratic (e.g., phenylbutazone)
Cyclic thrombocytopenia
Nutritional deficiency
  Folate
  Vitamin B_{12}
  Iron (rare)
Viral infections
  Influenza
  Rubella
  Infectious mononucleosis
  Thai hemorrhagic fever
  Dengue fever
  Others
Paroxysmal nocturnal hemoglobinuria
Hereditary disorders
  Wiskott-Aldrich syndrome
  May-Hegglin anomaly

Congenital causes
    Fanconi's anemia
    Amegakaryocytic thrombocytopenia with congenital malformations
    Congenital rubella or cytomegalovirus infection
    Maternal thiazide ingestion

Increased Destruction
Congenital—nonimmune
    Erythroblastosis fetalis
    Maternal preeclampsia
    Congenital viral infection
    Giant cavernous hemangioma
Congenital—immune
    Maternal drug ingestion
    Isoimmune neonatal thrombocytopenia
    Maternal autoimmune thrombocytopenic purpura
Acquired—nonimmune
    Infections
        Bacterial
            Sepsis
            Typhoid fever
        Viral
            Infectious mononucleosis
            Cytomegalovirus
            Herpes
        Malaria
        Rickettsial
            Rocky Mountain spotted fever
    Toxic shock syndrome
    Microangiopathic hemolytic anemia
        Disseminated intravascular coagulation
        Thrombotic thrombocytopenic purpura
        Hemolytic-uremic syndrome
        Vasculitis
    Drugs
    Extracorporeal circulation
    Anaphylaxis
Acquired—immune
    Drug-induced
        Quinine/quinidine
        Gold salts
        Heparin
        Thiazides
        Sulfonamides
        Indomethacin
        Others

Neoplasia-associated
  Lymphoproliferative disorders
  Solid tumors
Collagen-vascular disorders
  Systemic lupus erythematosus
  Rheumatoid arthritis
AIDS/HIV infection
Posttransfusion purpura
Idiopathic autoimmune thrombocytopenic purpura
  Acute
  Chronic
Sarcoidosis
Hashimoto's thyroiditis
Hyperthyroidism

Sequestration/Dilution
Hypersplenism
Hypothermia
Extracorporeal circulation
Massive blood transfusion

References
1. Aster RH: Thrombocytopenia Due to Diminished or Defective Platelet Production; Thrombocytopenia Due to Enhanced Platelet Destruction by Non-immunologic and Immunologic Mechanisms; Thrombocytopenia Due to Sequestration of Platelets; Thrombocytopenia Due to Platelet Loss. In general reference 18, pp 1343, 1351, 1370, 1398, 1401.
2. Aboulafia DM, Mitsuyasu RT: Hematologic Abnormalities in AIDS. *Hematol Oncol Clin N Am* 5:195, 1991.

8-K. Thrombocytosis

Primary
Myeloproliferative disorders
  Essential thrombocythemia
  Polycythemia vera
  Chronic myelogenous leukemia
  Agnogenic myeloid metaplasia with myelofibrosis

Secondary
Chronic inflammatory disorders
  Collagen-vascular disorders
    Rheumatoid arthritis
    Polyarteritis nodosa
    Wegener's granulomatosis
    Other vasculitis
  Chronic infections
    Tuberculosis
    Osteomyelitis
    Others
  Acute infections
  Inflammatory bowel disease
    Ulcerative colitis
    Regional ileitis
  Sarcoidosis
  Hepatic cirrhosis
Malignancy
Acute hemorrhage
Iron deficiency
Hemolytic anemia
Splenectomy
Recovery from thrombocytopenia (rebound)
  Myelosuppressive drug-induced
  Vitamin B_{12} or folate deficiency
  Alcohol-induced

Reference
1. Williams WJ: Thrombocytosis. In general reference 18, p 1403.

8-L. Pancytopenia

Aplastic anemias
  Congenital
    Fanconi's anemia
  Drug-/chemical-induced
    Benzene
    Chloramphenicol
    Phenylbutazone
    Gold salts
    Cytotoxic chemotherapy
    Alcohol
    Others
  Radiation exposure
  Idiopathic
  Infection
    Viral, especially hepatitis
  Immunologic
Hematologic neoplasia
  Leukemia (aleukemic)
  Lymphoproliferative disorders
    Lymphoma with marrow involvement
    Plasma cell myeloma
    Hairy-cell leukemia
  Myeloproliferative disorders
    Agnogenic myeloid metaplasia with myelofibrosis
  Myelodysplastic syndromes
Marrow infiltration/replacement
  Infection
    Tuberculosis
    Fungal
  Gaucher's and other lipid storage diseases
  Solid tumor
  Osteopetrosis
Nutritional deficiencies
  Vitamin B_{12}
  Folate
Other
  Collagen vascular diseases
    Systemic lupus erythematosus
  Paroxysmal nocturnal hemoglobinuria
  Hypersplenism
  Bacterial sepsis
  Viral infection
  AIDS/HIV infection
  Sarcoidosis

References
1. Williams DM: Pancytopenia, Aplastic Anemia, and Pure Red Cell Aplasia. In general reference 17, p 911.
2. Adamson JW, Erslev AJ: Aplastic Anemia. In general reference 18, p 158.

8-M. Lymphadenopathy

Benign
Infection
  Bacterial (any)
    Mycobacterial
  Fungal
  Viral
  Protozoal
  Rickettsial
  Chlamydial
Local inflammation
  Trauma
  Dermatitis
Hypersensitivity reaction
  Serum sickness
  Drug reaction
    Phenytoin
Collagen-vascular disorders
  Systemic lupus erythematosus
  Rheumatoid arthritis
  Dermatomyositis
Endocrine disorders
  Hyperthyroidism
AIDS/HIV infection
Sarcoidosis
Other
  Mucocutaneous lymph node syndrome
  Angioimmunoblastic lymphadenopathy
  Autoimmune hemolytic anemia

Malignant
Acute leukemia
Lymphoproliferative disorders
  Lymphoma
  Plasma cell myeloma
  Chronic lymphocytic leukemia
  Hairy-cell leukemia

Myeloproliferative disorders
   Chronic myelogenous leukemia
   Agnogenic myeloid metaplasia
Solid tumors

Reference

1. Williams WJ: Lymph Node Enlargement. In general reference 18, p 954.

8-N. Splenomegaly

Infection
   Bacterial
   Viral
   Rickettsial
   Fungal
   Protozoal
Inflammatory
   Collagen-vascular disorders
   Hypersensitivity reactions
      Serum sickness
      Drug reactions
Hematologic neoplasms
   Acute leukemia
   Lymphoproliferative disorders
      Lymphoma
      Chronic lymphocytic leukemia
      Hairy-cell leukemia
   Myeloproliferative diseases
   Myelodysplastic syndromes
Nonmalignant hematologic disorders
   Autoimmune hemolytic anemia
   Congenital hemolytic anemias
      Hemoglobinopathies
      Hereditary spherocytosis
   Megaloblastic anemias
   Iron-deficiency anemia
   Angioimmunoblastic lymphadenopathy
Congestive splenomegaly
   Portal hypertension
   Splenic or portal vein compression or thrombosis
   Congestive heart failure
   Budd-Chiari syndrome

Infiltrative disorders
   Gaucher's and other lipid storage diseases
   Histiocytic disorders
   Amyloidosis
   Metastatic solid tumors
Other
   AIDS/HIV infection
   Sarcoidosis
   Splenic trauma/hemorrhage
   Splenic cysts
   Splenic abscess

References
1. Athens JW: Disorders Primarily Involving the Spleen. In general reference 17, p 1704.
2. Jandl JH: The Spleen and Hypersplenism. In Jandl JH: *Blood: Textbook of Hematology.* Boston: Little, Brown, 1987, p 407.

8-O. Disorders of Hemostasis

Platelet Disorders
Quantitative platelet disorders (see 8-J)
Qualitative platelet disorders
   Congenital
      Bernard-Soulier syndrome
      Glanzmann's thrombasthenia
      Storage pool deficiencies
      Von Willebrand's disease
   Acquired
      Uremia
      Myeloproliferative disorders
      Myelodysplastic syndromes
      Dysproteinemias
      Drug-induced
         Aspirin
         Nonsteroidal antiinflammatory agents
         Dextran
         Hydroxyethyl starch
         Dipyridamole
         Sulfinpyrazone
         Others
      Extracorporeal circulation

Coagulation Disorders
Congenital
  Factor deficiencies
    VIII (hemophilia A)
    IX (hemophilia B)
    XI
    V
    VII
    X
    II
    Combined deficiency of vitamin K–dependent factors
  Fibrinogen disorders
    Afibrinogenemia
    Hypofibrinogenemia
    Dysfibrinogenemia
  Von Willebrand's disease
Acquired
  Vitamin K deficiency
    Malabsorption syndromes
    Broad-spectrum antibiotic therapy
    Cholestatic jaundice
    Dietary deficiency
    Hemorrhagic disease of the newborn
    Oral anticoagulant use/abuse
  Factor X deficiency and amyloidosis
  Circulating anticoagulants
    Factor VIII
      Associated with hemophilia A
      Autoimmune disorders
      Lymphoproliferative disorders/dysproteinemias
      Pregnancy
      Drug therapy
        Penicillin
    Factor IX and others
    Lupus anticoagulant
      With Factor II deficiency
  Consumptive coagulopathies
    Disseminated intravascular coagulation
  Liver disease
  Acquired dysfibrinogenemia
  Fibrinolytic states
  Heparin administration
  Massive blood transfusion

References
1. Bennett JS, Shattil SJ: Congenital Qualitative Platelet
   Disorders; Acquired Qualitative Platelet Disorders. In
   general reference 18, pp 1407, 1419.

2. Furie B: Disorders of the Vitamin K–dependent Coagulation Factors; Acquired Anticoagulants. In general reference 18, pp 1510, 1514.
3. Ratnoff OD, Forbes CD (eds): *Disorders of Hemostasis*. Philadelphia: Saunders, 1991.

8-P. Hypercoagulable States

Congenital
Antithrombin III deficiency
Protein C deficiency
Protein S deficiency
Homocystinuria
Dysfibrinogenemias

Acquired
Oral contraceptive use
Lupus anticoagulant
Myeloproliferative disorders
  Essential thrombocythemia
  Polycythemia vera
Paroxysmal nocturnal hemoglobinuria
Heparin-associated thrombocytopenia
Prothrombin complex concentrate infusion
Nephrotic syndrome
Pregnancy
Disseminated intravascular coagulation (DIC)
Thrombotic thrombocytopenic purpura
Malignancy (with DIC)
Sickle cell anemia
Hyperviscosity syndromes
Previous venous thrombosis
Venous trauma

References
1. Jandl JH: Thrombotic and Fibrinolytic Disorders. In Jandl JH (ed): *Blood: Textbook of Hematology*. Boston: Little, Brown, 1987, p 1141.
2. Schafer AI: The Hypercoagulable States. *Ann Intern Med* 102:814, 1985

8-Q. Disorders of Immunoglobulin Synthesis

Hypogammaglobulinemia
Congenital
  X-linked agammaglobulinemia
  Selective IgA deficiency
  Severe combined immunodeficiency
Acquired
  Common variable immunodeficiency
  Lymphoproliferative disorders
    Plasma cell myeloma
    Lymphoma
    Chronic lymphocytic leukemia
  Radiation therapy
  Antineoplastic chemotherapy
  Associated with thymoma

Hypergammaglobulinemia
Polyclonal
  Chronic inflammatory disease
    Chronic infections
    Collagen-vascular disorders
    Malignancy
    Hepatic cirrhosis
    Chronic active hepatitis
    AIDS/HIV infection
    Inflammatory bowel disease
    Sarcoidosis
    Others
  Angioimmunoblastic lymphadenopathy
Monoclonal
  Lymphoproliferative malignancies
    Plasma cell myeloma
    Non-Hodgkin's lymphoma
    Chronic lymphocytic leukemia
    Macroglobulinemia
    Heavy chain diseases
  Amyloidosis
  Monoclonal gammopathy of undetermined significance

References
1. Weinberg KI, Parkman R: Immunodeficiency Diseases. In general reference 18, p 967.
2. Bergsagel DE: Plasma Cell Neoplasms—General Considerations. In general reference 18, p 1101.

9 INFECTIOUS DISEASE

9-A. Fever of Unknown Origin in the United States*

Infection†
Bacterial
  Sinusitis
  Bacterial endocarditis
  Intravascular catheter infections
  Osteomyelitis
  Upper abdominal cause
    Cholangitis
    Cholecystitis
    Empyema of gallbladder
    Pancreatic, hepatic, splenic, subphrenic abscess
  Lower abdominal cause
    Appendiceal abscess
    Diverticulitis
    Pelvic inflammatory disease or abscess
    Perirectal abscess
    Peritonitis
  Urinary tract cause
    Perinephric, intrarenal, or prostatic abscess
    Pyelonephritis (rare)
    Ureteral obstruction

Acute rheumatic fever
Bacteremia without primary focus, especially:
  Meningococcemia
  Gonococcemia
  Salmonellosis
  Listeriosis
  Brucellosis
  Yersiniosis
  Tularemia
  Leptospirosis
  Syphilis
Tuberculosis
Viral (e.g., Epstein-Barr virus [infectious mononucleo-
    sis], hepatitis, Coxsackie B, cytomegalovirus,
    acquired immunodeficiency syndrome [AIDS]/HIV
    infection)
Chlamydial, rickettsial (e.g., psittacosis, Q fever)
Parasitic, protozoan, especially:
  Amebiasis
  Trichinosis
  Malaria
  Toxoplasmosis
Fungal, especially:
  Histoplasmosis
  Blastomycosis
  Cryptococcosis
  Coccidioidomycosis

Malignancy†
Leukemia, lymphoma
Solid tumor, especially carcinoma of:
  Kidney
  Lung
  Pancreas
  Liver
  Colon
Metastatic carcinoma
Atrial myxoma

Collagen-Vascular Disease†
Lupus erythematosus
Rheumatoid arthritis
Rheumatic fever
Polyarteritis nodosa, hypersensitivity vasculitis
Wegener's granulomatosis
Temporal arteritis
Kawasaki syndrome

Drugs
Antibiotics, especially:
  Penicillins
  Cephalosporins
  Sulfonamides
  Amphotericin B
Allopurinol
Phenytoin
Barbiturates
Iodides
Methyldopa
Procainamide
Quinidine
Propylthiouracil

Other
Pulmonary emboli, multiple
Thrombophlebitis
Sarcoidosis
Hepatitis, granulomatous or alcoholic
Inflammatory bowel disease
Whipple's disease
Thyroiditis
Thyrotoxicosis
Trauma with hematoma in enclosed space (e.g., peri-
  splenic, perivesical)
Myelofibrosis
Hemolytic states
Dissecting aneurysm
Fabry's disease
Familial Mediterranean fever
Gout
Addison's disease
Weber-Christian disease
Cyclic neutropenia
Thermoregulatory disorders
Factitious fever
Habitual hyperthermia

References
1. Petersdorf RG, Root RK: Chills and Fever. In general reference 1, p 125.
2. Jacoby GA, Swartz MN: Current Concepts: Fever of Undetermined Origin. N Engl J Med 289:1407, 1973.

*Defined as temperature of $> 38.3°C$ daily for 2 to 3 weeks, with cause undiagnosed despite 1 week of intensive studies in hospital.
†Infection, malignancy, and collagen-vascular disease ultimately account for about 75% of fevers of unknown origin.

9-B. Most Common Organisms Causing Specific Infections

Infection	Organisms
Skin infection	
Burns	*Staphylococcus aureus, Enterobacteriaceae, Pseudomonas sp., Serratia sp., Providencia sp., Aspergillus, herpes simplex, cytomegalovirus*
Decubiti	*S. aureus*; groups A, C, D, and anaerobic streptococci; *Enterobacteriaceae; Pseudomonas sp.; Bacteroides sp.*
Wounds (traumatic and surgical)	*S. aureus*, group A and anaerobic streptococci; *Enterobacteriaceae, Clostridium perfringens, Clostridium tetani*
Bites—Human	Viridans streptococci, group A streptococci, *S. aureus, Bacteroides sp., Staphylococcus epidermidis, Corynebacterium, Eikenella, Peptostreptococcus*
Bites—Cat	*Pasteurella multocida, S. aureus*
Bites—Dog	Viridans streptococci, *S. aureus, S. epidermidis, P. multocida, Bacteroides sp., Fusobacterium sp., Capnocytophaga*
Meningitis	Viruses, pneumococci, meningococci, group B and D streptococci, *Haemophilus influenzae, Enterobacteriaceae, Pseudomonas sp., Listeria monocytogenes* In HIV-infected patients: *Cryptococcus neoformans, Mycobacterium tuberculosis*, syphilis, and HIV aseptic meningitis

Otitis media	Pneumococci, *H. influenzae*, *Moraxella catarrhalis*, *S. aureus*, group A streptococci, *Enterobacteriaceae*
Conjunctivitis	Adenovirus, enterovirus, *H. influenzae*, pneumococci, *Neisseria*, *Chlamydia trachomatis*, coxsackievirus
Keratitis	*Pseudomonas* sp., pneumococci, *S. aureus*, *Neisseria gonorrhoeae*, *Neisseria meningitidis*, herpes simplex, fungi (*Fusarium*, *Aspergillus*, *Candida*), *Acanthamoeba* (associated with contact lens use)
Sinusitis	Pneumococci, *H. influenzae*, group A streptococci, anaerobes, viruses In diabetics: *Rhizopus* sp. (*Mucoraceae*), *Aspergillus*
Pharyngitis	Viruses; group A, C, and G streptococci; *Corynebacterium diphtheriae*; Epstein-Barr virus; gonococci; *Arcanobacterium hemolyticum*
Laryngitis Bronchitis	Respiratory viruses, group A streptococci, *M. catarrhalis*, *Chlamydia* sp. Respiratory syncytial virus, adenovirus, *Mycoplasma pneumoniae*, *Streptococcus pneumoniae*, *H. influenzae*, *M. catarrhalis*, staphylococci, *Chlamydia* sp., pertussis
Pneumonia	Respiratory viruses, *S. pneumoniae*, group A streptococci, *H. influenzae*, *Klebsiella* and other gram-negative bacilli, *S. aureus*, *M. pneumoniae*, *Legionella pneumophila* In HIV-infected patients: *P. carinii*, *M. tuberculosis*, histoplasmosis, Kaposi's sarcoma, coccidioidomycosis

9-B. Most Common Organisms Causing Specific Infections (continued)

Infection	Organisms
Lung abscess	*Bacteroides* sp., peptostreptococci, *Fusobacterium* sp., *Clostridium* sp.
Endocarditis	
Acute	*S. aureus, S. epidermidis*, pneumococci, group A and D streptococci, *Enterobacteriaceae*, diphtheroids, *C. albicans*, other fungi
Subacute	Viridans streptococci, *Streptococcus bovis*, enterococci, *Haemophilus parainfluenzae, Haemophilus aphrophilus*, fungi, especially *Candida* and *Aspergillus*
Septic thrombophlebitis	*S. aureus, S. epidermidis, Candida* sp., *Pseudomonas* sp., *Enterobacteriaceae*
Gastroenteritis	Enteric viruses, *Escherichia coli, Salmonella, Shigella, S. aureus, Campylobacter jejuni* In HIV-infected patients: *Cryptosporidium, Isospora belli*
Peritonitis	*Enterobacteriaceae*, enterococci, *Bacteroides*, group A streptococci, pneumococci, *S. aureus, Pseudomonas aeruginosa*
Urinary tract infections	
Cystitis, pyelonephritis	Herpes simplex, *Chlamydia trachomatis, Enterobacteriaceae, Staphylococcus saprophyticus*, gonococci, *Pseudomonas*, enterococci, *M. tuberculosis*

Urethritis	*C. trachomatis*, gonococci, Herpes simplex
Vaginitis	Viruses, *Chlamydia*, *Candida* sp., *Trichomonas*, *Gardnerella vaginalis*, *Bacteroides* sp.; peptococci, *Treponema pallidum*
Pelvic inflammatory disease—salpingitis	*N. gonorrhoeae*, *Chlamydia*, *Enterobacteriaceae*, *Bacteroides*, *Mycoplasma*, streptococci
Epididymitis—orchitis	*Enterobacteriaceae*, *N. gonorrhoeae*, *C. trachomatis*, *M. tuberculosis*
Prostatitis	*Enterobacteriaceae* (*E. coli*), *Pseudomonas*, gonococci, *S. aureus*, enterococci, *C. trachomatis*
Septicemia	*E. coli* and other gram-negative bacilli, *S. aureus*, *S. epidermidis*, pneumococci, groups A and D streptococci, *Bacteroides*
Osteomyelitis	*S. aureus*, group A, B streptococci; *Enterobacteriaceae*; *Pseudomonas* sp.; *Salmonella* sp., *H. influenzae*
Arthritis, septic	*S. aureus*; pneumococcus; group A, B streptococci; *H. influenzae*; gonococci; *S. epidermidis*; *Enterobacteriaceae*

References

1. General reference 19.
2. Sanford JP: *Guide to Antimicrobial Therapy 1993*. Dallas; Antimicrobial Therapy, Inc., 1993.

9-C. Antimicrobial Drugs of Choice

Organism	Drugs
GRAM-POSITIVE COCCI	
Staphylococcus aureus or *epidermidis*	Penicillin or penicillinase-resistant penicillin, cephalosporin, vancomycin, clindamycin, imipenem (add aminoglycoside for initial infective endocarditis therapy)
Streptococcus pneumoniae	Penicillin, cephalosporin, erythromycin, chloramphenicol, vancomycin
Streptococcus pyogenes (group A)	Penicillin, erythromycin, cephalosporin, clarithromycin
Enterococcus (group D streptococcus)	Ampicillin, amoxicillin, vancomycin (with gentamicin or amikacin)
Anaerobic streptococcus species	Penicillin G, clindamycin, erythromycin, vancomycin
GRAM-NEGATIVE COCCI	
Neisseria gonorrhoeae	Ceftriaxone, spectomycin, fluoroquinolones, penicillin G, amoxicillin with probenecid, trimethoprim/sulfamethoxazole (TMP/SMX)
Neisseria meningitidis	Penicillin G, cefotaxime, ceftriaxone (prophylaxis: rifampin, ciprofloxacin)
Moraxella (Branhamella) catarrhalis	TMP-SMX, amoxicillin-clavulanic acid, erythromycin, azithromycin
GRAM-POSITIVE BACILLI	
Bacillus anthracis (anthrax)	Penicillin G, ciprofloxacin, erythromycin, tetracycline
Clostridium difficile	Metronidazole or vancomycin orally, bacitracin
Clostridium perfringens	Penicillin G, chloramphenicol, metronidazole, clindamycin

Clostridium tetani	Penicillin G or a tetracycline; erythromycin
Listeria monocytogenes	Ampicillin with or without gentamicin, TMP/SMX, tetracycline, erythromycin, chloramphenicol, penicillin G
GRAM-NEGATIVE BACILLI	
Haemophilus influenzae	Cefotaxime or ceftriaxone (serious infections), TMP/SMX, ampicillin or amoxicillin, cefuroxime, tetracycline, clarithromycin, azithromycin
Escherichia coli	Cefotaxime, ceftizoxime, ceftriaxone, ceftazidime, ampicillin with or without aminoglycoside, ticarcillin, ampicillin-sulbactam, TMP/SMX
Helicobacter pylori	Tetracycline plus metronidazole plus bismuth subsalicylate
Klebsiella pneumoniae	Cefotaxime, ceftizoxime, ceftriaxone, ceftazidime, aminoglycoside, ciprofloxacin, aztreonam
Enterobacter	Imipenem, cefotaxime, ceftizoxime, aminoglycoside, ticarcillin, aztreonam, fluoroquinolone
Proteus mirabilis	Ampicillin, cephalosporin, ticarcillin, aminoglycoside, imipenem
Providencia stuartii	Cefotaxime, imipenem, ticarcillin-clavulanic acid, aminoglycoside, aztreonam, fluoroquinolone
Serratia	Cefotaxime, ceftizoxime, ceftriaxone, ceftazidime, gentamicin, imipenem, TMP/SMX, aztreonam, fluoroquinolones
Pseudomonas aeruginosa	Ciprofloxacin (UTI), ticarcillin plus tobramycin, ceftazidime, imipenem
Salmonella typhi	Ceftriaxone, chloramphenicol, ampicillin, amoxicillin, TMP/SMX, fluoroquinolone
Shigella	Fluoroquinolone, TMP/SMX, ampicillin, ceftriaxone

9-C. Antimicrobial Drugs of Choice *(continued)*

Organism	Drugs
Bacteroides	
Oropharyngeal	Penicillin G, clindamycin, cefoxitin
Gastrointestinal	Metronidazole, clindamycin, imipenem
Brucella	Tetracycline plus gentamicin; chloramphenicol, with or without streptomycin; TMP/SMX
Bordetella pertussis	Erythromycin, TMP/SMX, ampicillin
Acinetobacter	Imipenem, aminoglycoside, ticarcillin
Legionella pneumophila	Erythromycin plus rifampin, TMP/SMX, clarithromycin, azithromycin, ciprofloxacin
MISCELLANEOUS	
Mycobacterium tuberculosis	Isoniazid, with rifampin; pyrazinamide, with or without ethambutol
Mycobacterium avium	Clarithromycin, rifampin, ethambutol, clofazimine, ciprofloxacin
Actinomyces israelii	Penicillin G, tetracycline
Nocardia	TMP/SMX, sulfisoxazole, amikacin, imipenem
Treponema pallidum	Penicillin G, tetracycline, ceftriaxone
Leptospira	Penicillin G, tetracycline
Mycoplasma pneumoniae	Erythromycin, tetracycline, clarithromycin
Rickettsia	Tetracycline, chloramphenicol, fluoroquinolone
Chlamydia trachomatis	Tetracycline, erythromycin, ofloxacin

Pneumocystis carinii	TMP/SMX, pentamidine
Toxoplasma gondii	Pyrimethamine and sulfonamide
Giardia lamblia	Quinacrine, metronidazole, furazolidone
Trichomonas vaginalis	Metronidazole

FUNGI

Aspergillus	Amphotericin B, flucytosine
Blastomyces dermatitidis	Ketoconazole, amphotericin B
Candida albicans	Amphotericin B with or without flucytosine and rifampin (topical: amphotericin B, clotrimazole, econazole, miconazole, nystatin)
Coccidioides immitis	Ketoconazole, amphotericin B (meningitis)
Cryptococcus neoformans	Ketoconazole, amphotericin B, flucytosine, fluconazole
Histoplasma capsulatum	Ketoconazole, amphotericin B
Sporothrix schenchii	Potassium iodide (topical), amphotericin B

VIRUSES

Herpes simplex	Acyclovir, ganciclovir; acyclovir-resistant herpes simplex virus: foscarnet; keratitis: trifluridine
HIV infection	Zidovudine (retrovir or azidothymidine [AZT]), didanosine (DDI), dideoxycytidine (DDC)
Influenza A	Amantadine
Respiratory syncytial virus	Ribavirin
Varicella zoster	Acyclovir, vidarabine
Cytomegalovirus (CMV) pneumonia	Ganciclovir

References
1. General reference 19.
2. The Choice of Antimicrobial Drugs. *Med Let,* 28(710):33, 1992.
3. Sanford JP: *Guide to Antimicrobial Therapy 1993.* Dallas; Antimicrobial Therapy, Inc., 1993.
4. Peiperi, L. *Manual of HIV/AIDS Therapy: Current Clinical Strategies.* Newport Beach, CA: Publishing International, 1992.
5. Jong, E. *The Travel and Tropical Medicine Manual.* Philadelphia: Saunders, 1987.

9-D. CDC HIV Classification System

Clinical Category A
Asymptomatic HIV infection
Persistent generalized lymphadenopathy (nodes in 2 or more extrainguinal sites, at least 1 cm in diameter for 3 months or more)
Acute (primary) HIV illness

Clinical Category B*
Bacterial endocarditis, meningitis, pneumonia, sepsis
Candidiasis, vulvovaginal, persisting more than 1 month
Candidiasis, oropharyngeal
Cervical dysplasia, severe or carcinoma
Constitutional symptoms, e.g., fever (38.5° C) or diarrhea lasting more than 1 month
Hairy leukoplakia, oral
Herpes zoster, 2 or more episodes or more than 1 dermatome
Idiopathic thrombocytopenic purpura
Listeriosis
Mycobacterium tuberculosis, pulmonary
Pelvic inflammatory disease
Peripheral neuropathy

Clinical Category C
Candidiasis; esophageal, tracheal, bronchial
Coccidiodomycosis, extrapulmonary
Cryptococcosis, extrapulmonary
Cryptosporidiosis, chronic intestinal (< 1 mo)
Cytomegalovirus retinitis, or other than liver or spleen nodes

HIV encephalopathy
Herpes simplex with mucocutaneous ulcer for more than 1 month, bronchitis, pneumonia
Isosporiasis, chronic, lasting more than 1 month

Kaposi's sarcoma
Lymphoma: Burkitt's, immunoblastic, primary in brain

Mycobacterium avium or Mycobacterium kansasii, extrapulmonary
M. tuberculosis, extrapulmonary
Mycobacterium, other species disseminated or extrapulmonary
Pneumocystis carinii pneumonia
Progressive multifocal leukoencephalopathy
Salmonella bacteremia, recurrent
Toxoplasmosis, cerebral
Wasting syndrome due to HIV

1993 Revised CDC HIV classification system

	Clinical category		
CD4 cell category	A	B	C
≥ 500/mm^3	A1	B1	C1
200–499/mm^3	A2	B2	C2
< 200/mm^3	A3	B3	C3

Note: Categories A3, B3, C1, C2, C3 comprise the expanded CDC clinical definition of AIDS.
Source: Adapted from Centers for Disease Control: 1993 Revised Classification System for HIV Infection and Expanded Surveillance Case Definition for AIDS Among Adolescents and Adults. *MMWR* 41(RR-17):1–19, 1992.

References
1. Centers for Disease Control. Revision of the CDC Surveillance Case Definition for Acquired Immunodeficiency Syndrome. *MMWR* 1987;26:3S–15S.
2. Centers for Disease Control. 1993 Revised Classification System for HIV Infection and Expanded Surveillance Case Definition for AIDS Among Adolescents and Adults. *MMWR* 1992;41(RR-17):1–19.

*Must be attributed to HIV infection or have a clinical course or management complicated by HIV.

9-E. VDRL, Biologic False-Positive

Infection
Spirochetal
  Yaws
  Pinta
  Bejel
  Leptospirosis
  Relapsing fever
  Rat-bite fever
Bacterial
  Pneumococcal pneumonia
  Scarlet fever
  Subacute bacterial endocarditis
  Tuberculosis
  Leprosy
  Chancroid
Viral
  Measles
  Varicella
  Vaccinia
  Hepatitis
  Infectious mononucleosis
  Postimmunization
Mycosplasmal
Chlamydial (lymphogranuloma venereum)
Rickettsial (typhus)
Protozoal (malaria, sleeping sickness)
Filarial
Fungal (coccidioidomycosis)

Noninfectious Causes
Aging
Pregnancy
Drug addiction
Collagen-vascular disease (especially lupus erythematosus, rheumatoid arthritis)
Serum sickness
Thyroiditis
Other hypergammaglobulinemic states
Blood transfusion
Malignancy

References
1. Rudolph A: Syphilis. In general reference 19, p 623.
2. Lukehart SA, Holmes KK: Syphilis. In general reference 1, p 657.

10 INTEGUMENT

10-A. Alopecia

Nonscarring

Aging (pattern baldness)
Androgenetic alopecia (e.g., secondary to ovarian or adrenal dysfunction)
Traction or other trauma (trichotillomania, heat exposure)
Drugs
    Cytotoxic agents
    Oral contraceptives (withdrawal)
    Amphetamines
    Heparin
    Warfarin
    Beta blockers
    Levodopa
    Lithium
    Bromocriptine
    Thallium
    Bismuth
    Borax
    Vitamin A, retinoids
    Ethionamide
    Propylthiouracil
Serious systemic illness, childbirth, other stresses (telogen effluvium)

Cutaneous disease
  Seborrheic dermatitis
  Eczema
  Tinea capitis
  Psoriasis
  Cosmetics, other local irritants
Lupus erythematosus
Hypothyroidism
Hypopituitarism
Syphilis, secondary
Nutritional deficiency states (kwashiorkor, marasmus; iron, zinc, biotin deficiency)
Alopecia areata
Hereditary
Congenital

Scarring
Physical and chemical agents
  Burns
  Freezing
  Mechanical trauma
  Acid, alkali
  Radiation
Infection
  Bacterial (including pyogenic infection, tertiary syphilis, leprosy, lupus vulgaris)
  Fungal (e.g., ringworm)
  Viral (especially varicella-zoster, variola)
  Protozoal (leishmaniasis)
Systemic disease
  Lupus erythematosus, systemic or discoid
  Scleroderma or morphea
  Sarcoidosis
  Dermatomyositis
  Amyloidosis
  Neoplasm
    Metastatic carcinoma
    Lymphoma
Cutaneous disease
  Basal cell carcinoma
  Lichen planus
  Cicatricial pemphigoid
  Necrobiosis lipoidica diabeticorum
  Folliculitis decalvans
  Pseudopelade
Congenital

References
1. Bertolino AP, Freedberg IM: Hair. In general reference
   20, p 627.
2. General reference 1.

10-B. Erythema Multiforme

Infections
    Viral (especially herpes simplex, Epstein-Barr, cox-
      sackie)
    Bacterial (e.g., *Yersinia, Francisella tularensis*)
    Mycoplasmal
    Chlamydial (lymphogranuloma venereum)
    Fungal (especially histoplasmosis, coccidioidomycosis)
    Parasitic (*Trichomonas,* malaria)
Vaccines (e.g., smallpox, polio, bacille Calmette-Guérin
    [BCG])
Drugs, toxins
    Antibiotics (especially penicillin, sulfonamides, tetracy-
      clines, ethosuximide)
    Metals: arsenic, mercury, gold
    Antihistamines
    Barbiturates
    Codeine
    Phenytoin
    Carbamazepine
    Sulfonylureas
    Codeine
    Hydralazine
    Salicylates
    Thiazides
    Phenylbutazone
    Phenolphthalein
Neoplasms and hematologic disorders
    Lymphoma
    Leukemia
    Carcinoma
    Multiple myeloma
    Polycythemia vera
Physical factors and contact reactions
    Radiation
    Sunlight
    Cold

Poison oak
Fire sponge (*Tedania ignis*)
Collagen-vascular disease
  Lupus erythematosus, systemic or discoid
  Rheumatoid arthritis
  Polyarteritis nodosa
  Wegener's granulomatosis
  Dermatomyositis
  Reiter's syndrome
Sarcoidosis
Menstruation, pregnancy
Loeffler's syndrome
Beer ingestion
Idiopathic

Reference

1. Elias PM, Fritsch PO: Erythema Multiforme. In general reference 20, p 555.

10-C. Erythema Nodosum

Infection
  Bacterial
    Streptococci
    Yersinia
    Cat-scratch fever
    Tularemia
  Fungal
    Histoplasmosis
    Coccidioidomycosis
    Blastomycosis
    Trichophyton
  Tuberculosis
  Leprosy
  Leptospirosis
  Chlamydial (lymphogranuloma venereum, psittacosis)
  Viral
Drugs
  Penicillins
  Sulfonamides
  Salicylates
  Halides
  Oral contraceptives

Sarcoidosis
Behçet's syndrome
Leukemia, lymphoma
Radiation therapy
Inflammatory bowel disease
Idiopathic

Reference
1. Bordi EE, Lazarus GS: Panniculitis. In general reference
    20, p 1131.

10-D. Hirsutism and Generalized Hypertrichosis

Anorexia, malnutrition
Drugs
   Minoxidil
   Corticosteroids
   Androgenic steroids
   Progestins
   Danazol
   Phenytoin
   Diazoxide
   Penicillamine
Endocrine disorders
   Adrenogenital syndrome
   Adrenal hyperplasia, adenoma, carcinoma
   Pituitary tumor (especially Cushing's disease, acromeg-
      aly, prolactin-secreting tumor)
   Polycystic ovary syndrome
   Ovarian tumor
   Hypothyroidism
Central nervous system disease
   Encephalitis
   Multiple sclerosis
   Head trauma
Dermatomyositis
Hereditary or congenital conditions
   Cutaneous porphyria
   Hurler's syndrome
   Morquio's disease
   Leprechaunism
   de Lange's syndrome
   Hypertrichosis lanuginosa

Reference
1. Bertolino AP, Freedberg IM: Hair. In general reference
   20, p 627.

10-E. Maculopapular Eruption, Generalized

Drugs (especially antibiotics)
Infections
  Viral
    Rubeola
    Rubella
    Roseola
    Erythema infectiosum (human parvovirus)
    Infectious mononucleosis
    Cytomegalovirus
    Hepatitis B
    Other viruses (including adeno-, entero-, reo-, arbo-,
      rhabdovirus)
    Live-virus vaccine (e.g., measles)
  Bacterial, especially:
    Streptococcal
    Staphylococcal
    Salmonella
    Meningococcemia, chronic
  Other
    Mycoplasmal
    Syphilis, secondary
    Leptospirosis
    Rat-bite fever
    Rickettsial (e.g., Rocky Mountain spotted fever, murine
      typhus)
    Psittacosis
    Toxoplasmosis
    Trichinosis
Systemic lupus erythematosus
Dermatomyositis
Sarcoidosis
Pityriasis rosea

Reference
1. General reference 20.

10-F. Petechiae and Purpura

Platelet Disorders
Thrombocytopenia (see 8-J)
  Drugs, especially:
    Cytotoxic agents
    Aspirin
    Phenytoin
    Nonsteroidal antiinflammatory agents
    Quinidine
    Quinine
    Gold
  Disseminated intravascular coagulation
    Overwhelming infection
      Bacterial (especially meningococcal, gonococcal, staphylococcal, gram-negative)
      Viral (especially entero-, arbo-, adenovirus; acquired immunodeficiency syndrome [AIDS])
      Rickettsial (Rocky Mountain spotted fever, louse-borne typhus)
      Miliary tuberculosis
      Malaria
    Anaphylaxis
    Neoplasm (especially leukemia, lymphoma, and carcinoma of lung, prostate, or pancreas)
  Thrombotic thrombocytopenic purpura
  Immune thrombocytopenic purpura
  Posttransfusion purpura
  Wiskott-Aldrich syndrome
Functional platelet disorders (e.g., Glanzmann's thrombasthenia, von Willebrand's disease)
Thrombocytosis

Vascular/Extravascular Causes
Vasculitis (palpable purpura)
  Henoch-Schönlein purpura
  Polyarteritis nodosa
  Wegener's granulomatosis
  Lupus erythematosus
  Rheumatoid arthritis
  Subacute bacterial endocarditis
  Hepatitis B
  Serum sickness
  Cryoglobulinemia
  Sjögren's syndrome
  Hyperglobulinemic purpura
  Waldenström's macroglobulinemia

Lymphoproliferative disorders (especially Hodgkin's disease, lymphosarcoma)
Drugs
  Antibiotics (penicillin, sulfonamides, tetracycline)
  Thiazides
  Nonsteroidal antiinflammatory agents
  Hydralazine
  Cimetidine
  Phenytoin
  Allopurinol
  Quinidine
  Propylthiouracil
  Ketoconazole
  Gold
Aging
Prolonged elevated venous pressure or other trauma
Steroids (endogenous or exogenous)
Amyloidosis
Cholesterol embolization
Ehlers-Danlos syndrome
Pseudoxanthoma elasticum
Hereditary hemorrhagic telangiectasia
Scurvy
Progressive pigmentary purpura

Reference

1. Brodin MB, Zucker-Franklin D: The Skin and the Hematopoietic System. In general reference 20, p 1909.

10-G. Pruritus

Pruritus with Diagnostic Skin Lesions
Infestation (especially scabies, lice, fleas)
Xerosis (dry skin; e.g., secondary to low humidity or excessive bathing)
Infection, especially bacterial, fungal, varicella
Eczematous dermatitis (e.g., atopic, contact)
Urticaria (see 10-J)
Psoriasis
Dermatitis herpetiformis
Bullous pemphigoid
Lichen planus
Miliaria
Mastocytosis
Mycosis fungoides

Pruritus Without Diagnostic Skin Lesions
Infestation, especially:
  Hookworm
  Onchocerciasis
  Ascariasis
  Trichinosis
Drugs
  Opiates
  Aspirin
  Estrogens, progestins, androgens
  Erythromycin
  Sulfonylureas
  Phenothiazines
  Quinidine
  Vitamin B complex
  Psoralen/ultraviolet A radiation (PUVA)
Obstructive liver disease
  Bile duct obstruction, extrahepatic
  Bile duct obstruction, intrahepatic
    Biliary cirrhosis
    Drug-induced cholestasis (oral contraceptives, phenothiazines, chlorpropamide)
    Intrahepatic cholestasis of pregnancy
Neoplasm, especially:
  Lymphoma, leukemia
  Abdominal malignancy
  Central nervous system malignancy
  Carcinoid tumor
Polycythemia vera
Iron deficiency

Diabetes mellitus
Hyperthyroidism
Chronic renal failure (with or without secondary hyperparathyroidism)

Reference
1. Bernhard JD: Clinical Aspects of Pruritus. In general reference 20, p 78.

10-H. Pustules, Generalized

Acne vulgaris
Pyogenic infection (especially disseminated gonococcal)
Viral infection (especially vaccinia, variola)
Syphilis, secondary
Drugs, especially:
 Sulfonamides
 Phenytoin
 Halides
 Corticosteroids
 Androgenic steroids
 Oral contraceptives
Pustular psoriasis
Sweet's syndrome (acute febrile neutrophilic dermatosis)
Behcet's syndrome

Reference
1. General reference 20.

10-I. Telangiectasia

Normal variant (especially with wind or sun exposure)
Endocrine disease
   Chronic liver disease (especially alcoholic cirrhosis)
   Pregnancy, estrogen, or progesterone therapy
   Topical steroid therapy (long-term)
   Hyperthyroidism
Collagen-vascular disease
   Lupus erythematosus, systemic or discoid
   Dermatomyositis
   Rheumatoid arthritis
   Systemic sclerosis, CRST syndrome
Genetically transmitted disease
   Osler-Rendu-Weber syndrome (hereditary hemorrhagic
     telangiectasia)
   Ataxia-telangiectasia
   Fabry's disease
   Xeroderma pigmentosum
States associated with prolonged vasodilatation (e.g., vari-
   cose veins, rosacea, polycythemia vera)
Peripheral vascular disease (e.g., livedo reticularis, ery-
   thema ab igne)
Neoplastic disease, especially:
   Breast cancer
   Bile duct carcinoma
   Carcinoid tumor
   Malignant angioendotheliomatosis
Radiation dermatitis

Reference
1. General reference 20.

10-J. Urticaria

Specific antigen sensitivity (e.g., foods, Hymenoptera
  venom, helminths)
Physical agents
  Pressure, mechanical irritation
  Cold
  Heat
  Light (e.g., sunlight)
Atopic conditions (e.g., allergic rhinitis, asthma)
Drugs
  Opiates, barbiturates
  Antibiotics (especially penicillin, sulfonamides)
  X-ray contrast media
  Nonsteroidal antiinflammatory agents
  Azo dyes
  Curare
Transfusion of blood or blood components
Vasculitis
  Lupus erythematosus
  Rheumatoid arthritis
  Sjögren's syndrome
  Serum sickness
  Hepatitis B, acute
  Cryoglobulinemia
Mastocytosis (urticaria pigmentosa)
Occult malignancy (especially lymphoma, carcinoma)
Emotional stress
Idiopathic

Reference
1. Soter NA, Wasserman SI: IgE-dependent Urticaria and
   Angioedema. In general reference 20, p 1282.

10-K. Vesicles and Bullae, Generalized

Physical agents
    Radiation
    Burns
    Chemicals
    Mechanical irritation, trauma
Drugs
    Barbiturates
    Penicillins
    Sulfonamides
    Nitrofurantoin
    Nalidixic acid
    Thiazides
    Furosemide
    Nonsteroidal antiinflammatory agents
    Phenytoin
    Mephenytoin
    Allopurinol
    Phenolphthalein
Infections
    Bacterial
        Disseminated gonococcus, *Pseudomonas*
        Impetigo, erysipelas
        Toxic epidermal necrolysis
        Staphylococcal scalded skin syndrome
    Viral
        Herpes simplex
        Herpes zoster
        Varicella
        Variola (smallpox)
        Vaccinia
        Enterovirus (e.g., hand-foot-mouth disease)
    Syphilis, congenital
    Rickettsialpox
Erythema multiforme bullosum, Stevens-Johnson syn-
      drome (see 10-B)
Pemphigus
Pemphigoid
Acute eczematous dermatitis, especially contact dermatitis
Dermatitis herpetiformis
Epidermolysis bullosa
Porphyria
Lupus erythematosus, discoid or systemic
Pityriasis rosea (vesicular type)
Diabetes mellitus

Herpes gestationis
Subcorneal pustular dermatosis
Bullous ichthyosis

Reference

1. Section 11: Epidermis: Disorders of Dermal and Dermal-Epidermal Cohesion—Vesicular and Bullous Disorders. In general reference 20, p 546.

11 MUSCULO-SKELETAL SYSTEM

11-A. Shoulder Pain

Fracture
Contusion
Acromial-clavicular joint separation/injuries
Rotator cuff tendinitis/impingement syndrome
Bursitis
Bicipital tendinitis (long head)
Referred pain
  Diaphragmatic irritation
    Biliary disease
    Blood or gas in peritoneal or pleural cavity
    Subphrenic abscess
    Splenic trauma
    Neoplasm
    Lower-lobe pleuropulmonary inflammatory disease
  Apical lung cancer (Pancoast syndrome)
  Cervical radiculopathy/brachial neuritis
  Angina pectoris and/or myocardial infarction
Osteoarthritis
Infectious arthritis
Rheumatoid arthritis
Crystalline arthritis
Arthritis associated with collagen-vascular disease
Rupture of rotator cuff

Anterior/posterior shoulder instability
Shoulder-hand syndrome
Neoplasm, primary or metastatic
Local arterial, venous, or lymphatic occlusion
Adhesive capsulitis
Thoracic outlet syndromes
    Cervical and first-rib syndromes, scalenus anterior syndrome
    Hyperabduction syndrome
    Costoclavicular syndrome
Myalgias and arthralgias
Fibrositis syndromes
Psychogenic pain
Sleep dysesthesias
Congenital/developmental abnormalities
Postural

References

1. Thornhill, T: The Painful Shoulder. In general reference 21, p 491.
2. Schumacher HR (ed): *Primer on the Rheumatic Diseases* (9th ed). Atlanta: Arthritis Foundation, 1988.
3. Neviaser RJ (ed): Management of Shoulder Problems. *Orthop Clin North Am* 18(3), 1987.

11-B. Back Pain

Functional, mechanical causes: postural imbalance
    Anteroposterior (e.g., pregnancy)
    Lateral (e.g., scoliosis, unequal leg lengths)
Trauma
    Lumbar strain or sprain
    Lumbosacral disk herniation
    Vertebral fracture (compression or other)
    Subluxation of facet joints
Osteoarthritis, spondylosis
Rheumatoid arthritis
Fibromyalgia
Polymyalgia rheumatica
Spondylitis and/or sacroiliitis
    Ankylosing spondylitis
    Colitic (enteropathic) spondylitis
    Psoriatic arthritis
    Behçet's syndrome
    Reiter's syndrome

Familial Mediterranean fever
Syphilis
Ochronosis
Spinal stenosis
  Congenital
  Degenerative
  Iatrogenic (post-laminectomy/-fusion/-chemonucleolysis)
  Posttraumatic
  Paget's disease
  Fluorosis
Spinal or vertebral tumor
  Benign (e.g., hemangioma, meningioma, osteoid osteoma)
  Malignant
    Primary (e.g., multiple myeloma, ependymoma, osteogenic sarcoma)
    Metastatic, especially:
      Prostate
      Non-Hodgkin's lymphoma, Hodgkin's lymphoma
      Breast
      Leukemic
      Lung
      Kidney
      Thyroid
      Gastrointestinal tract
Infection (e.g., disk space infection, vertebral osteomyelitis, epidural abscess)
  Bacteria (usually secondary to hematogenous spread)
  Brucella
  Spirochetes
  Parasites
  Herpes zoster
  Mycobacteria
  Fungi
Congenital causes
  Facet tropism
  Transitional vertebrae
  Spina bifida
  Spondylolysis, spondylolisthesis
Hyperparathyroidism
Osteomalacia (e.g., vitamin D–resistant rickets)
Osteoporosis (primary, endocrine, nutritional, drug)
Scheuermann's disease (epiphysitis)
Radium poisoning
Osteogenesis imperfecta
Referred pain
  Vascular disease (especially abdominal aortic aneurysm, Leriche syndrome)

Hip pain
  Pelvic or prostatic inflammation or tumor, endometriosis
  Retroperitoneal hematoma or tumor
  Renal disease
    Stone
    Infection
    Tumor
    Polycystic kidney disease
  Abdominal disease (e.g., intestinal, pancreatic, gall-
    bladder)
  Cardiorespiratory (pulmonary emboli, pleuritis, coronary
    ischemia, pneumonitis)
Hematologic disorders
  Hemoglobinopathies (e.g., sickle cell, myelofibrosis)
Psychoneurotic causes
  Hysteria
  Malingering

References
1. Mankin H: Back and Neck Pain. In general reference 1,
   pp 118–122.
2. Wiesel S, et al: The Current Approach to the Medical Diagnosis of Low Back Pain. *Orthop Clin North Am*
   22(2):315, 1991.

11-C. Myalgias

Fibrositis
Connective-tissue disease
  Polymyalgia rheumatica
  Rheumatoid arthritis
  Polymyositis, dermatomyositis
  Lupus erythematosus
  Polyarteritis nodosa
  Scleroderma
Systemic infection, especially:
  Viral illness
    Influenza
    Coxsackievirus infection
    Arbovirus infection
    Hepatitis
    Rabies
    Poliomyelitis
  Rheumatic fever
  Salmonellosis

 Tularemia
 Brucellosis
 Glanders
 Trichinosis
 Leptospirosis
 Relapsing fever
 Malaria
Rhabdomyolysis (see 11-D)
Drugs (e.g., amphotericin B, clofibrate, carbenoxolone)
Hypothyroidism
Hyperparathyroidism
Hypoglycemic myopathy
Congenital enzyme deficiency (e.g., phosphorylase [Mc-
  Ardle's disease], phosphofructokinase)
Polyneuropathy (e.g., Guillain-Barré disease)
Ischemic atherosclerotic disease (i.e., intermittent claudica-
  tion)

Reference
1. Part 13, Section 2: Diseases of Nerve and Muscle. In
 general reference 1, p 2088.

11-D. Muscle Weakness

Acute or Subacute*
Electrolyte abnormality
 Hyperkalemia
 Hypokalemia
 Hypercalcemia
 Hypermagnesemia
 Hypophosphatemia
Rhabdomyolysis
 Extreme muscular exertion
 Prolonged seizures
 Hyperthermia
 Extensive crush injury or muscle infarction
 Influenza
 Hypokalemia
 Hypophosphatemia
 Alcoholic myopathy
 Snake venoms
 Industrial toxin ingestion
 Familial myoglobinuria
 Metabolic myopathies (e.g., McArdle's disease)
Polymyositis, dermatomyositis

Infection, especially:
  Viral
    Influenza
    Coxsackievirus infection
    Rabies
    Poliomyelitis
    Herpes zoster
  Trichinosis
  Toxoplasmosis
  Botulism
  Diphtheria
  Leprosy
  Cysticercosis
  Schistosomiasis
  Trypanosomiasis
  Landry-Guillain-Barré-Strohl syndrome
Peripheral neuropathy, acute (see 12-Q)
Thyrotoxicosis
Corticosteroid therapy
Organophosphorus poisoning

Chronic
Progressive muscular dystrophy, especially:
  Duchenne's
  Facioscapulohumeral
  Limb-girdle
  Myotonic
Endocrine disorders
  Hyperthyroidism or hypothyroidism
  Hyperparathyroidism
  Vitamin D deficiency (e.g., vitamin D–deficiency rickets)
  Corticosteroid therapy
  Cushing's syndrome/Addison's disease
  Acromegaly
Connective-tissue disease
  Lupus erythematosus
  Rheumatoid arthritis
  Polymyositis, dermatomyositis
  Sjögren's syndrome
  Mixed connective-tissue disease
Alcoholic myopathy
Chronic polymyopathy
  Glycogen storage disease
  Central core disease
  McArdle's disease
  Familial periodic paralysis with progressive myopathy
Progressive neural-muscular atrophy
  Amyotrophic lateral sclerosis

Multiple sclerosis
Werdnig-Hoffman disease
Peroneal muscular atrophy (Charcot-Marie-Tooth disease)
Chronic peripheral neuropathy (e.g., arsenic, lead, nutritional; see also 12-Q)

Intermittent and/or Transient
Electrolyte abnormality
Hypokalemia
Hyperkalemia
Hypophosphatemia
Hypercalcemia
Hypermagnesemia
Hyperkalemic or hypokalemic periodic paralysis
Drugs
Aminoglycosides (especially neomycin, streptomycin, kanamycin, polymyxin B)
Steroids
Vincristine
Chloroquine
Bretylium
Clofibrate
Myasthenia gravis
Eaton-Lambert syndrome
Acute thyrotoxic myopathy
Thyrotoxic periodic paralysis
Paramyotonia congenita
Adynamia episodica hereditaria

References
1. Part 13, Section 2: Diseases of Nerve and Muscle. In general reference 1, p 2088.
2. Miller M, Phelps P: Weakness. In general reference 21, p 462.

*Developing over days to weeks. See also Intermittent and/or Transient.

11-E. Polyarticular Arthritis

Rheumatoid arthritis*
Juvenile rheumatoid arthritis*
Rheumatic fever*
Ankylosing spondylitis*
Collagen-vascular diseases
  Lupus erythematosus*
  Scleroderma*
  Polymyositis, dermatomyositis*
  Mixed connective-tissue disease
  Polyarteritis nodosa (rare)*
  Henoch-Schönlein purpura (rare)*
  Wegener's granulomatosis (rare)*
  Other vasculitides (rare; e.g., allergic granulomatosis)*
  Polymyalgia rheumatica*
Immunologically mediated diseases
  Serum sickness*
  Hyperglobulinemic purpura*
  Hypogammaglobulinemia*
  Mixed cryoglobulinemia (rare)*
Systemic diseases
  Sjögren's syndrome*
  Reiter's syndrome*
  Psoriasis*
  Behçet's syndrome*
  Inflammatory bowel disease*
    Ulcerative colitis
    Regional enteritis
  Intestinal bypass*
  Pancreatic disease
    Carcinoma
    Pancreatitis
  Whipple's disease*
  Familial Mediterranean fever*
  Amyloidosis
  Sarcoidosis*
  Hematologic disorders
    Leukemia*
    Lymphoma*
    Multiple myeloma*
    Hemophilia
    Hemoglobinopathies (especially sickle cell anemia, thalassemia)*

Storage diseases (e.g., Gaucher's disease, Fabry's disease, hyperlipoproteinemia)*
  Ochronosis
  Hemochromatosis
  Wilson's disease
  Acromegaly
  Hypothyroidism
  Renal transplantation
Degenerative joint disease
Trauma
Neuropathic arthropathy (e.g., tabes dorsalis, diabetes mellitus, syringomyelia)
Joint tumor
  Pigmented villonodular synovitis
  Hemangioma
  Sarcoma
Infection*
  Bacterial (especially gonococcus, staphylococcus, pneumococcus)
  Viral (especially hepatitis B, mumps, rubella, arboviruses, parvovirus, retrovirus)
  Tuberculous
  Fungal (candida with central venous line/hyperalimentation)
  Rickettsial
  Parasitic
  Lyme disease
Others
  Gout*
  Pseudogout*
  Hypertrophic osteoarthropathy
  Intermittent hydrarthrosis*
  Palindromic rheumatism*
  Radiation
  Relapsing polychondritis*
  Acute tropical polyarthritis*
  Tietze's syndrome
Nonarticular rheumatism
  Bursitis*
  Periarthritis*
  Tendinitis*
  Tenosynovitis*
  Epicondylitis
  Myositis
  Fibrositis
  Fasciitis

References
1. General reference 21.
2. Bennett JC: Infectious Etiology of Rheumatoid Arthritis. *Arthritis Rheum* 21:531, 1978.

*Usually inflammatory (i.e., joints painful, swollen, stiff, often erythematous and warm).

11-F. Monoarticular (Oligoarticular) Arthritis

Juvenile rheumatoid arthritis
Ankylosing spondylitis
Rheumatoid arthritis (rare)
Systemic diseases
  Psoriasis
  Behçet's syndrome
  Inflammatory bowel disease (ulcerative colitis, regional
    enteritis)
  Pancreatic disease (carcinoma, pancreatitis)
  Whipple's disease
  Familial Mediterranean fever
  Hematologic disorders
    Leukemia
    Lymphoma
    Bleeding-clotting disorders (hemophilia, von Wille-
      brand's disease, anticoagulant use)
    Hemoglobinopathies (especially sickle cell anemia,
      thalassemia)
  Storage diseases (e.g., Gaucher's, Fabry's)
  Acromegaly
  Amyloidosis
Degenerative joint disease
Trauma
Neuropathic arthropathy (e.g., tabes dorsalis, diabetes mel-
  litus, syringomyelia)
Joint tumors (e.g., pigmented villonodular synovitis, hem-
  angioma, sarcoma)
Infection
  Bacterial (especially gonococcus, staphylococcus, pneu-
    mococcus)
  Viral (especially hepatitis B, rubella, mumps)
  Tuberculous
  Fungal

Rickettsial
Parasitic
Others
  Gout
  Pseudogout
  Intermittent hydrarthrosis
  Loose joint body
  Foreign body
  Palindromic rheumatism
  Radiation
  Relapsing polychondritis
Nonarticular rheumatism
  Bursitis
  Periarthritis
  Tendinitis
  Tenosynovitis
  Epicondylitis
  Myositis
  Fibrositis
  Fasciitis

Reference

1. McCune WJ: Monoarticular Arthritis. In general reference 21, p 442.

11-G. Characteristics of Synovial Fluid

	Normal	Noninflammatory	Inflammatory	Purulent	Hemorrhagic
Color	Clear to pale yellow	Xanthochromic	Xanthochromic to white	White	
Clarity	Transparent	Transparent	Translucent to opaque	Opaque	
Viscosity	High	High	Low	Low*	
Mucin clot	Good	Good to fair	Fair to poor	Poor	
Spontaneous clot	None	Often	Often	Often	
WBCs/mm³	< 150	< 3000	3000–50,000	> 50,000	
% Polymorphs	< 25	< 25	> 70	> 90	
Glucose (mg/dl)	Nearly equal to blood	Nearly equal to blood	> 25, lower than blood	> 50, lower than blood	
Culture	Negative	Negative	Negative	Often positive	
Conditions in which findings are likely to occur		Osteoarthritis Trauma Neuropathic arthropathy	Rheumatoid arthritis Connective tissue diseases (SLE, PSS, DM/PM)	Bacterial arthritis Tuberculous arthritis	Trauma Anticoagulation Neuropathic arthrop-

Chronic or subacute crystal synovitis
SLE
Scleroderma
Polymyalgia rheumatica
Erythema nodosum
Polyarteritis nodosa
Amyloidosis

Viral arthritis
Ankylosing spondylitis
Seronegative spondyloarthropathies (Reiter's syndrome, psoriatic arthritis, inflammatory bowel disease arthritis)
Acute gout or pseudogout
Rheumatic fever
Behçet's syndrome

athy: Charcot joints
Joint tumor (pigmented villonodular synovitis or hemangioma)
Hematologic disorders (especially hemophilia, sickle cell trait or disease)
Joint prosthesis

SLE = systemic lupus erythematosus; PSS = progressive systemic sclerosis; DM/PM = dermatomyositis/polymyositis.

*May be high in infection with coagulase-positive staphylococcus.

Source: Group designations from Ropes MW, Bauer W: Synovial Fluid Changes in Joint Diseases. Cambridge, Mass.: Harvard University Press, 1953. Table modified from McCarty DJ, McCarty WJ (eds): Arthritis and Allied Conditions (12th ed). Philadelphia: Lea & Febiger, 1993, pp 64–65. and from Schumacher HR (ed): Primer on Rheumatic Diseases (9th ed). Atlanta: Arthritis Foundation, 1988, pp 55–60.

11-H. Clubbing

Usually with Hypertrophic Osteoarthropathy
Neoplasm
  Intrathoracic
    Lung
    Pleura
    Mediastinum (Hodgkin's disease)
    Thymus
  Esophagus, stomach
  Intestine
  Liver
Other pulmonary disorders
  Lung abscess
  Empyema
  Chronic pneumonitis
  Pneumoconiosis
  Bronchiectasis
  Tuberculosis
  Cystic fibrosis
Idiopathic, hereditary (pachydermoperiostitis)

Usually Without Hypertrophic Osteoarthropathy
Genetic
Subacute bacterial endocarditis
Cyanotic congenital heart disease
Chronic liver disease (e.g., biliary cirrhosis)
Intestinal disorders
  Ulcerative colitis
  Regional enteritis
  Sprue, steatorrhea
  Bacterial or amebic dysentery
  Tuberculosis, intestinal
Hyperparathyroidism
Graves' disease (thyroid acropachy)
Occupational trauma (e.g., jackhammer operation)

Unilateral
Aneurysm of aorta or of subclavian, innominate, or brachial
  artery
Shoulder subluxation
Hemiplegia
Axillary or apical lung tumor

Unidigital
Median nerve injury

Sarcoidosis
Tophaceous gout

Reference
1. Altman RD, Tenenbaum J: Hypertrophic Osteoarthropathy. In general reference 21, p 1666.

11-I. Raynaud's Phenomenon

Raynaud's disease
Chronic arterial disease
    Atherosclerosis
    Thromboangiitis obliterans
    Thrombosis
    Embolism
Pulmonary venoocclusive disease
Collagen-vascular disease
    Scleroderma
    Lupus erythematosus
    Rheumatoid arthritis
    Polyarteritis nodosa
    Mixed connective-tissue disease
    Polymyositis, dermatomyositis
    Sjögren's syndrome
Occupational exposure
    Vibration (e.g., pneumatic tools)
    Percussion (e.g., typing)
    Vinyl chloride polymerization
Drugs, toxins
    Heavy metals (lead, arsenic, thallium)
    Methysergide, ergot compounds
    Beta-adrenergic blockers
    Chemotherapy (bleomycin, vinblastine)
Hematologic disorders
    Dysproteinemias (e.g., multiple myeloma, Waldenström's macroglobulinemia)
    Polycythemia vera, essential thrombocythemia
    Leukemia
    Cryoglobulinemia
    Cold agglutinin phenomenon
Neurologic disorders
    Peripheral neuropathy
    Hemiplegia
    Intervertebral disk herniation

    Spinal cord tumor
    Multiple sclerosis
    Transverse myelitis
    Syringomyelia
Carpal tunnel syndrome
Thoracic outlet syndrome
Posttraumatic reflex sympathetic dystrophy
Post–cold injury (e.g., frostbite)
Acromegaly
Myxedema
Fabry's disease

References
1. General reference 1.
2. Seibold JR: Scleroderma. In general reference 21,
   p 1222.

11-J. Osteomalacia

Vitamin D deficiency
    Dietary deficiency
    Insufficient sun exposure
    Malabsorption (e.g., pancreatic insufficiency, small-intes-
       tine disease, postgastrectomy)
Disordered vitamin D metabolism (hereditary or acquired)
    Chronic renal failure
    Anticonvulsant therapy
    Chronic liver disease (e.g., biliary cirrhosis)
Peripheral resistance to vitamin D (e.g., vitamin D–depen-
    dent rickets)
Chronic acidosis (e.g., distal renal tubular acidosis, chronic
    acetazolamide ingestion, ureterosigmoidostomy)
Phosphate depletion (see 1-O)
Impaired renal tubular phosphate resorption
    Vitamin D–resistant rickets
    Fanconi syndrome (hereditary or acquired)
    Tumor phosphaturia
    Neurofibromatosis
    Neonatal (transient)
    Intoxications (cadmium, lead, outdated tetracycline, alu-
       minum)
Miscellaneous
    Osteopetrosis
    Hypophosphatasia
    Fluorosis

Magnesium-dependent conditions
Parenteral hyperalimentation
Renal transplantation
Tumor-associated renal disease

References

1. Singer F: Metabolic Bone Disease. In Feliz P, et al: *Endocrinology and Metabolism.* New York: McGraw-Hill, 1987, p 1458.
2. Krane SM, Holick MF: Metabolic Bone Disease. In general reference 1, p 1921.

11-K. Osteopenia*

Aging (especially postmenopause)†
Immobilization
Nutritional causes
  Calcium and/or vitamin D deficiency
  Malnutrition, malabsorption
  Postgastrectomy
  Scurvy
Corticosteroid excess
  Cushing's syndrome or disease
  Steroid therapy
Other endocrine disorders
  Hypogonadism (e.g., Klinefelter's syndrome, Turner's
    syndrome, early oophorectomy)
  Thyrotoxicosis
  Acromegaly
  Hyperparathyroidism
  Hypopituitarism
  Diabetes mellitus
Inherited bone matrix abnormalities
  Homocystinuria
  Marfan's syndrome
  Ehlers-Danlos syndrome
  Osteogenesis imperfecta
  Menkes' syndrome
Rheumatoid arthritis
Ankylosing spondylitis
Malignancy, especially:
  Lymphoma
  Leukemia
  Multiple myeloma
  Waldenström's macroglobulinemia

Systemic mastocytosis
Carcinomatosis
Heparin therapy (chronic)†
Chronic obstructive pulmonary disease†
Chronic acidosis (especially renal tubular acidosis, metabolic acidosis secondary to high-protein diet)
Alcoholism
Hepatic insufficiency, cirrhosis (alcoholic or other)
Methotrexate†
Chronic anticonvulsant therapy
Chronic renal failure (renal osteodystrophy)
Paget's disease (with predominantly lytic lesions)
Juvenile (idiopathic)†
Cystic fibrosis†
Riley-Day syndrome
Menkes' syndrome
Down's syndrome
Hypophosphatasia, adult variety
Female distance runners
Smoking

References
1. Singer F: Metabolic Bone Disease. In Feliz P, et al: *Endocrinology and Metabolism.* New York: McGraw-Hill, 1987, p 1468.
2. Riggs BL, Melton LJ: The Prevention and Treatment of Osteoporosis. *N Engl J Med* 327:9, 1992.

*Decreased bone mass.
†Characterized on bone biopsy by decreased bone mass with normal mineral-to-matrix ratio.

11-L. Antibodies to Nuclear or Cytoplasmic Antigens

Disease	Antibodies most commonly associated
Systemic lupus erythematosus	Antinative (double-stranded) DNA
	Anti–single-stranded DNA
	Antiribonucleoprotein (anti-RNP)
	Anti-Sm
	Anti-Ro/SSA
	Anti-La/SSB
	Antihistone (especially drug-induced lupus)
Progressive systemic sclerosis	Antinucleolar
	Anticentromere
	Anti-Scl-70 (especially in scleroderma/polymyositis overlap syndrome)
	Anti-RNP
Polymyositis/ scleroderma overlap syndrome	Anti-Jo-1
	Anti-Ku-1
	Anti-PM-1
Mixed connective tissue disease	Anti-RNP
Sjögren's syndrome	Anti-Ro/SSA
	Anti-La/SSB

References
1. McCarty DJ, McCarty WJ (eds); *Arthritis and Allied Conditions* (12th ed). Philadelphia: Lea & Febiger, 1993, p 1182.
2. Schumacher HR (ed): *Primer on Rheumatic Diseases* (9th ed). Atlanta: Arthritis Foundation, 1988, p 35.
3. Reichlin M: Significance of Ro Antigen System. *J Clin Immunol* 6(5):339, 1986.

11-M. Rheumatoid Factor

Aging
Rheumatoid arthritis
Systemic lupus erythematosus
Progressive systemic sclerosis
Dermatomyositis, polymyositis
Infections
   Syphilis
   Influenza
   Subacute bacterial endocarditis
   Infectious mononucleosis
   Bacterial bronchitis
   Viral hepatitis
   Tuberculosis
   Leprosy
   Parasitic infection (e.g., schistosomiasis, kala-azar)
   Following extensive immunizations
   Lyme disease
   Acquired immune deficiency syndrome (AIDS)
   Cytomegalovirus
   Rubella
   Periodontal disease
Sjögren's syndrome (with or without arthritis)
Chronic active hepatitis and cirrhosis
Lymphoma
Waldenström's macroglobulinemia
Mixed cryoglobulinemia
Hypergammaglobulinemic purpura
Chronic lung disease
   Pneumoconiosis (e.g., silicosis, asbestosis)
   Sarcoidosis
   Interstitial fibrosis, idiopathic
Multiple transfusions
Renal transplantation

References
1. Lipsky PE: Rheumatoid Arthritis. In general reference 1, p 1437.
2. McCarty DJ, McCarty WJ (eds): *Arthritis and Allied Conditions* (12th ed). Philadelphia: Lea & Febiger, 1993, p 871.

11-N. Systemic Lupus Erythematosus Criteria*

Facial erythema (butterfly rash)
Discoid lupus erythematosus
Photosensitivity
Nonerosive arthritis
Oral or nasopharyngeal ulceration
Serositis (pleuritis and/or pericarditis)
Psychosis and/or seizures
Proteinuria > 0.5 gm/day or cellular casts in urine (red cell,
    hemoglobin, granular, tubular, mixed)
Hematologic disorder:
   Hemolytic anemia, leukopenia (WBC < 4000/mm^3),
    lymphopenia (< 1500/mm^3), or thrombocytopenia
    (< 100,000/mm^3)
Antinuclear antibody
Immunologic disorder: positive LE cell preparation, anti-
    DNA antibodies, anti-Sm antibodies, or chronic false-
    positive serologic test for syphilis

Diagnosis of systemic lupus can be made if 4 or more of the above
11 criteria are present, serially or simultaneously, during any interval
of observation.
*Source: Tan EM, et al: The 1982 Revised Criteria for the Classifica-
tion of Systemic Lupus Erythematosus (SLE). *Arthritis Rheum*
25:1271, 1982.

12 NERVOUS SYSTEM

12-A. Dizziness and Vertigo

Dizziness
Hyperventilation
Anxiety, psychosomatic causes
Hypoxia
Anemia
Hypotension (especially orthostatic)
Hypertension
Cardiac arrhythmia
Peripheral neuropathy
Myelopathy
Concussion
Aging

True Vertigo
Infection
    Labyrinthitis (bacterial, viral, syphilitic)
    Cholesteatoma
    Chronic otitis media with middle-ear fistula
    Vestibular neuronitis/neuropathy
    Herpes zoster oticus
Vascular disorders
    Vertebrobasilar insufficiency or occlusion

Labyrinthine or internal auditory artery occlusion or spasm
Migraine
Hemorrhage into labyrinthine system, brainstem, or cerebellum (e.g., secondary to bleeding diathesis, leukemia, hypertension)
Ménière's disease
Benign positional vertigo of Bárány
Drugs and toxins
  Alcohol
  Quinine
  Aminoglycoside antibiotics (especially streptomycin, gentamicin)
  Salicylates
  Benzene
  Arsenic
  Arsine
Trauma
  Temporal bone fracture
  Labyrinthine concussion
  Postsurgical (inner-ear area)
  Perilymphatic fistula
Tumor, especially:
  Acoustic neuroma
  Epidermoid carcinoma
  Metastatic carcinoma (especially breast, kidney, lung, stomach)
  Glomus body tumor
Other
  Cerumen impaction
  Motion sickness
  Multiple sclerosis
  Extraocular muscle palsy
  Syringobulbia
  Tabes dorsalis
  Friedreich's ataxia
  Encephalitis
  Seizure aura

References

1. Haymaker W, Kuhlenbeck H: Disorders of the Brainstem and Its Cranial Nerves. In general reference 23, vol 3, chap 40.
2. Baloh RW: Neurotology. In general reference 23, vol 3, chap 42.
3. General reference 22, p 226.

12-B. Headache

Muscle contraction (tension)
Migraine
Cluster (histamine) headache
Nonmigrainous vascular causes
  Effort (physical activity)
  Vasomotor rhinitis
  Fever
  Hypertension
  Hypotension
  Hypoxia and/or hypercapnia (e.g., chronic obstructive
     pulmonary disease, pulmonary infiltrative disease,
     sleep apnea syndrome, high altitude)
  Anemia
  Cerebrovascular disease (thrombosis, embolism, hemor-
     rhage)
  Postseizure
  Post–lumbar puncture
  Endocrine causes
    Hypoglycemia
    Hypothyroidism
    Hyperthyroidism
    Adrenal insufficiency
    Carcinoid, serotonin-secreting tumors
    Premenstrual syndrome
Drugs and toxins
  Theophylline
  Caffeine and caffeine withdrawal
  Nitrates
  Nitrites (e.g., hot dogs)
  Dextroamphetamines
  Ephedrine
  Reserpine
  Monamine oxidase inhibitors plus catecholamines
  Monosodium glutamate (MSG)
  Histamine
  Steroid withdrawal
  Alcohol withdrawal
  Disulfiram (Antabuse) plus alcohol
  Lead
  Benzene
  Carbon monoxide
  Carbon tetrachloride
  Insecticides
Intracranial causes
  Tumor

Arteriovenous malformation
Aneurysm (with or without hemorrhage)
Subdural hematoma
Encephalitis, brain abscess
Pseudotumor cerebri
Posttraumatic
Cranial inflammation
  Meningeal irritation/inflammation
    Infection (e.g., bacterial, viral, tuberculous, fungal)
    Carcinomatous infiltration
  Postsubarachnoid hemorrhage
  Vasculitis (e.g., temporal arteritis, lupus, polyarteritis nodosa)
Cranial and neck causes
  Sinuses (trauma, inflammation)
  Ears (external, middle, internal)
  Eyes (inflammation, trauma, increased intraocular pressure, poor refraction)
  Teeth, jaws (infection, trauma, temporomandibular joint malocclusion)
  Cervical spine, ligaments, muscles (trauma, cervical spondylosis, ankylosing spondylitis, tumor)
  Neuralgia (e.g., postherpetic, trigeminal, glossopharyngeal)
Psychogenic, psychiatric

References
1. Ziegler DK, Murrow RW: Headache. In general reference 23, vol 2, chap 13.
2. General reference 22, p 134.

12-C. Paresthesias

Peripheral neuropathy (see 12-Q), especially associated
    with:
  Diabetes mellitus
  Alcoholism
  Thiamine deficiency
Peripheral nerve entrapment, compression, trauma (e.g.,
    intervertebral disk herniation, thoracic duct outlet syn-
    drome, carpal tunnel syndrome)
Atherosclerotic peripheral vascular disease
Spinal cord disease
  Spinal cord or nerve root compression
  Multiple sclerosis
  Tabes dorsalis
  Subacute combined degeneration of spinal cord (perni-
    cious anemia, vitamin B_{12} deficiency)
  Strachan's syndrome
Metabolic disturbance
  Hypocalcemia
  Respiratory alkalosis

References
1. General reference 1.
2. General reference 22.

12-D. Syncope

Neurological and/or Mechanical Causes

- Mediated by vagal stimulation and/or autonomic insufficiency
  - Vasovagal reaction (often associated with strong emotion or pain)

  Prolonged recumbency or inactivity

  Peripheral neuropathy with autonomic involvement (e.g., diabetes, amyloidosis, tabes dorsalis)

  Drugs (e.g., nitrates, antihypertensive agents, ganglionic blockers, alcohol)
  - Carotid sinus syncope
  - Micturition syncope
  - Swallow syncope
  - Bowel stimulation/defecation syncope

  Airway stimulation (e.g., suctioning)
  - Eyeball pressure

  Glossopharyngeal neuralgia

  Sympathectomy

  Neuro Primary autonomic insufficiency
- Seizure   { *Basilar Artery insufficiency   ∈ TIA , CVA*

  Head trauma   (*vertebral-basilar ˮ*)

  Reduced cardiac output/venous return

  Hypovolemia

  Hypotension

  Valsalva maneuver

  Cough

  Voluntary forced expiration against closed glottis

  Weight lifting

  Atrial myxoma or thrombus

  Cardiac tamponade

Atherosclerosisofcarotid   Carotid steal syn

Cardiopulmonary Causes   *CV : ↓BP   Atrialmyxoma*
- Cardiac arrhythmias (see 2-O)   *orthrombus*

  Bradyarrhythmias (e.g., sick sinus syndrome)

  Tachyarrhythmias (especially ventricular fibrillation, ventricular tachycardia, paroxysmal atrial tachycardia)

  Atrioventricular block

  Pulmonary embolism
- Myocardial infarction with cardiogenic shock
- Pericardial tamponade
- Aortic stenosis

  Pulmonic stenosis

  Primary pulmonary hypertension

pul: emboli . pul stenosis PPH

Cerebrovascular Causes
- Atherosclerotic disease of carotid and/or cerebral vessels (especially vertebral-basilar insufficiency)

  Takayasu's arteritis

  Hypertensive encephalopathy

  Cervical spine abnormalities (e.g., cervical spondylosis)

Metabolic Causes
- Anemia *hypovolemia*
- Hypoxia
- Hyperventilation
- Hypoglycemia *Dm*

Drug: nitrate,
antihypertensive
agent
alcohol

Psychological Causes
- Anxiety, hysteria

References
1. General reference 22, p 291.
2. Johnson RH, Lambie DG, Spalding JMK: The Autonomic Nervous System. In general reference 23, vol 4, chap 57.

12-E. Deafness

Sensorineural (Inner Ear)
Aging

Prolonged exposure to loud noise

Drugs

  Salicylates

  Aminoglycoside antibiotics (especially neomycin, amika-cin)

  Furosemide, ethacrynic acid

  Quinine

  Cisplatin

Infection

  Chronic middle or inner ear infection

  Cholesteatoma

  Labyrinthitis

    Bacterial

    Viral (e.g., mumps)

    Syphilis (usually congenital)

  Herpes zoster oticus

Autoimmune disease (e.g., polyarteritis nodosa, Cogan's syndrome)

Ménière's disease

Tumor of eighth nerve or cerebellopontine angle (especially
acoustic neuroma)
Eighth nerve infarction
Multiple sclerosis
Hereditary or congenital causes (e.g., congenital rubella,
Alport's syndrome)

Conductive

Cerumen impaction
Otosclerosis
Chronic otitis media, cholesteatoma
Trauma (including temporal bone fracture, bleeding into
middle ear)
Mucopolysaccharidoses

References

1. General reference 22, p 226.
2. Baloh RW: Neurotology. In general reference 23, vol 3,
chap 42.

12-F. Ataxia

Cerebellar Disease (Cerebellar Ataxia)

Alcoholic cerebellar degeneration, Wernicke's disease
Degenerative or demyelinating disease (e.g., multiple scle-
rosis, Huntington's chorea)
Neoplasm or paraneoplastic cerebellar degeneration
Vascular occlusion or hemorrhage (vertebral-basilar arter-
ies or branches)
Vasculitis (e.g., systemic lupus erythematosus, polyarteritis
nodosa)
Seizure disorder (especially ataxic myoclonia)
Infection (encephalitis, meningitis, abscess)
Infiltrative disease (e.g., Hand-Schuller-Christian disease,
sarcoidosis)
Cranial trauma
Hypoglycemia
Posthyperthermia, heat stroke
Hypoxic encephalopathy
Drugs (e.g., phenytoin, barbiturates, carbamazepine)
Toxins (e.g., arsenic, lead, mercury, thallium, toluene, or-
ganophosphates)
Nonwilsonian hepatocerebral degeneration (posthepatic
coma)
Hypoparathyroidism

Congenital cerebellar anomalies (e.g., Dandy-Walker syndrome, Arnold-Chiari malformation)
Hereditary diseases (e.g., phenylketonuria, ataxia-telangiectasia, lipid storage disease, Machado-Joseph disease)
Primary cerebellar ataxias (e.g., olivopontocerebellar atrophy, corticocerebellar atrophy, dentate cerebellar atrophy)

Loss of Postural or Proprioceptive Sense (Sensory Ataxia)

Infection (e.g., neurosyphilis)
Endocrine disease (e.g., diabetes mellitus)
Toxins (e.g., arsenic, ergot)
Nutritional diseases
  Alcoholism
  Beriberi
  Pellagra
  Vitamin B_{12} deficiency
  Scurvy
Hereditary disease (e.g., Friedreich's ataxia, Refsum's disease)
Congenital
Other
  Multiple sclerosis
  Amyotrophic lateral sclerosis
  Primary posterolateral sclerosis
  Spinal cord tumor or compression

References

1. Dow RS, Kramer RE, Robertson LT: Diseases of the Cerebellum. In general reference 23, vol 3, chap 37.
2. General reference 22.

12-G. Acute Confusional State*

Delirium†
Drug withdrawal after chronic intoxication, especially:
  Alcohol
  Barbiturates
  Other sedatives
Drug intoxication, especially:
  Atropine
  Amphetamines
  Bromides
  Caffeine
  Camphor
  Ergot
  Scopolamine
Infectious and febrile illness, especially:
  Septicemia
  Pneumonia
  Typhoid fever
  Rheumatic fever
Central nervous system disorders
  Cerebrovascular disease (especially involving parietal or
    temporal lobes or upper brainstem)
  Brain tumor
  Encephalitis (especially viral)
  Meningitis
  Subarachnoid hemorrhage
  Head trauma (e.g., concussion, subdural hematoma)
  Postseizures
Thyrotoxicosis
Steroid psychosis (rare)

Other Acute Confusional States‡
Metabolic causes
  Electrolyte disorders, especially:
    Hyponatremia
    Hypercalcemia
    Hypokalemia
  Hypoxia
  Hypercarbia
  Congestive heart failure
  Hypoglycemia
  Hepatic encephalopathy
  Uremia
  Hypothyroidism
  Wernicke's disease
  Porphyria

Drug intoxication
  Barbiturates
  Narcotics
  Bromides
  Antihypertensive agents
Central nervous system disease
  Cerebrovascular disease (see 12-N)
  Brain tumor
  Brain abscess
  Meningitis
  Encephalitis
  Migraine
  Subdural or epidural hematoma
Febrile illness
Acute psychosis (e.g., postoperative, postpartum)
Preexisting dementia with superimposed stress (e.g., Alzheimer's, serious illness; see 12-H)

Reference
1. General reference 22, p 323.

*See also 12-H and 12-M.
†An acute, transient confusional state characterized by mental alertness, gross disorientation, hallucinations, psychomotor and autonomic hyperactivity.
‡Confusional states not associated with psychomotor or autonomic hyperactivity.

12-H. Dementia*

Degenerative diseases
  Senile dementia
  Alzheimer's disease
  Cerebral arteriosclerosis, multiple cerebrovascular accidents
  Pick's disease (circumscribed cerebral atrophy)
  Parkinson's disease
  Korsakoff's psychosis
  Demyelinating disease (e.g., multiple sclerosis, Schilder's disease [diffuse cerebral sclerosis])
  Amyotrophic lateral sclerosis
  Progressive supranuclear palsy (Steele-Richardson-Olszewski syndrome)
Metabolic causes
  Hypoxic encephalopathy
  Hypoglycemia
  Hypocalcemia (e.g., hypoparathyroidism)
  Hepatocerebral degeneration (posthepatic coma)
  Pernicious anemia, subacute combined degeneration of the spinal cord
  Pellagra
  Myxedema
  Cushing's disease
  Barbiturate intoxication, chronic
  Bromide intoxication
  Dialysis dementia
Infectious causes
  Brain abscess
  Chronic meningoencephalitis (e.g., cryptococcosis, neurosyphilis)
  Viral encephalitis (especially herpes simplex)
  Acquired immunodeficiency syndrome (AIDS)
  Progressive multifocal leukoencephalopathy
  Creutzfeldt-Jakob disease
Intracranial tumor
Head trauma (e.g., contusion, hemorrhage, subdural hematoma)
Myoclonic epilepsy
Normal-pressure hydrocephalus
Hereditary diseases
  Huntington's chorea
  Wilson's disease
  Lipid storage diseases (e.g., Tay-Sachs, leukodystrophies)
  Mucopolysaccharidoses

Pseudodementias
  Depression
  Hypomania
  Schizophrenia
  Hysteria

Reference
1. General reference 22, p 323.

*Deterioration of intellectual and cognitive functions with little or no disturbance of consciousness or perception. See also 12-G and 12-M.

12-I. Tremor

Tremor at rest (present at rest, decreased with movement)
  Parkinson's disease
  Postencephalitic parkinsonism
  Wilson's disease
  Phenothiazines (tardive dyskinesia)
  Brain tumor
Action tremor (present with movement, decreased at rest)
  Physiologic (anxiety, fatigue)
  Essential (senile and/or familial)
  Withdrawal from alcohol or opiates
  Meningoencephalitis (e.g., viral, paretic neurosyphilis)
  Hyperthyroidism
  Pheochromocytoma
  Carcinoid syndrome
  Bronchodilators, beta agonists
  Xanthines (e.g., coffee, tea)
  Steroids
  Lithium
Ataxic (increased at terminal phase of voluntary movement; see 12-F)

Reference
1. General reference 22, p 78.

12-J. Choreoathetosis

Hereditary diseases, especially:
  Wilson's disease
  Huntington's disease
  Lesch-Nyhan disease
  Lipid storage disease (e.g., Niemann-Pick)
  Dystonia musculorum deformans
Drugs
  Phenothiazines
  Haloperidol
  L-Dopa
  Dihydroxyphenylalanine
  Bromocriptine
Postinfectious (Sydenham's chorea)
  Rheumatic fever
  Diphtheria
  Rubella
  Pertussis
Pregnancy (chorea gravidarum)
Hypoxic encephalopathy
Kernicterus
Perinatal hypoxia or injury
Hyperthyroidism
Nonwilsonian hepatocerebral degeneration (posthepatic
  coma)
Lupus erythematosus
Acute disseminated encephalomyelitis (postinfectious,
  postvaccinal)
Corticostriatospinal degeneration
Thalamic infarct or hemorrhage

References
1. McDowell FH, Cedarbaum JM: The Extrapyramidal System and Disorders of Movement. In general reference 23, vol 3, chap 38.
2. General reference 22.

12-K. Nystagmus

Pendular*
Congenital
Spasmus nutans
Associated with bilateral central loss of vision before 2
    years of age
  Albinism
  Aniridia
  Bilateral chorioretinitis
  Congenital cataracts
  Corneal scarring
  Optic atrophy
Multiple sclerosis
Prolonged work in dim light (miner's nystagmus)

Jerk†
Nonpathologic
  Extreme lateral gaze
  Attempt to fix on moving objects (opticokinetic nystag-
    mus)
  Labyrinthine stimulation (e.g., cold water in auditory ca-
    nal)
Drugs
  Barbiturates
  Alcohol
  Phenytoin
  Phenothiazines
  Meperidine
Labyrinthine-vestibular disease (see 12-A)
Cerebellar lesions (e.g., Wernicke's disease, cerebellopon-
    tine angle tumor)
Encephalitis
Vascular disease involving brainstem (especially hyperten-
    sive infarction, posterior-inferior cerebellar artery occlu-
    sion)
Demyelinating disease (e.g., multiple sclerosis)
Brainstem tumor
Syringobulbia
Meningioma, meningeal cyst
Arnold-Chiari malformation
Congenital

Reference
1. General reference 22, p 206.

*Both components equal.
†Fast and slow components.

12-L. Seizures

Central Nervous System and Vascular Causes
Cerebrovascular disease (see 12-N)
  Thrombosis
  Embolism
  Hemorrhage (intracerebral or subarachnoid)
  Vasculitis (especially lupus erythematosus, polyarteritis nodosa, mixed connective tissue disease)
  Infarction
  Thrombophlebitis
  Arteriovenous malformation
Brain tumor (especially metastatic tumor, meningioma, astrocytoma)
Cerebral infection
  Encephalitis
  Meningitis (especially bacterial)
  Brain abscess
  Neurosyphilis
  Creutzfeldt-Jakob disease
Head trauma
Hypoxic encephalopathy
Reduced cerebral blood flow (e.g., hypotension, Stokes-Adams syndrome, carotid sinus syncope)
Hypertensive encephalopathy
Eclampsia
Alzheimer's disease
Pick's disease

Metabolic Causes
Fever
Alcohol withdrawal
Barbiturate withdrawal
Drugs, toxins
  Amphetamines
  Heroin
  Cocaine
  Phenothiazines
  Tricyclic antidepressants
  Lidocaine
  Aminophylline
  Salicylates
  Ergot
  Digitalis

Penicillins
Nalidixic acid
Isoniazid
Cycloserine
Physostigmine, other anticholinergics
Vincristine
Lithium
Lead
Mercury
Arsenic
Thallium
Strychnine
Camphor
Hypoglycemia
Hyperglycemia
Hyponatremia
Hypernatremia (or rapid correction of hypernatremia)
Hypocalcemia
Hypomagnesemia
Alkalosis (respiratory or metabolic)
Uremia
Dialysis dysequilibrium
Hepatic failure
Reye's syndrome
Thyrotoxicosis
Hypothyroidism
Pyridoxine deficiency
Pellagra

Congenital or Inherited Diseases
Congenital infection
  Toxoplasmosis
  Cytomegalovirus
  Syphilis
  Rubella (maternal)
Neonatal hypoxia or trauma, kernicterus
Down's syndrome
Lipid storage disease (e.g., Gaucher's disease)
Tuberous sclerosis
Sturge-Weber disease
Phenylketonuria
Acute intermittent porphyria

Idiopathic

References
1. General reference 22, p 249.
2. Forster FM, Booker HE: The Epilepsies and Convulsive Disorders. In general reference 23, vol 3, chap 31.

12-M. Coma*

Primary neurologic disease
    Cerebrovascular accident (thrombosis, embolism, hemorrhage—see 12-N), especially involving upper brainstem
    Hypertensive encephalopathy
    Head trauma
    Intracranial neoplasm
    Seizures and postictal state
    Meningitis, encephalitis, brain abscess
    Other
        Demyelinating disease (e.g., multiple sclerosis, central pontine myelinolysis, Schilder's disease)
        Creutzfeldt-Jakob disease
        Progressive multifocal leukoencephalopathy
        Marchiafava-Bignami disease
Metabolic causes
    Drugs, especially:
        Barbiturates
        Benzodiazepines
        Anesthetics
        Phenothiazines
        Narcotics
        Alcohol
    Toxins (e.g., methanol, carbon monoxide)
    Hypoxia
    Hypercapnia
    Shock (e.g., septic, cardiogenic; see 2-K)
    Acidosis, metabolic or respiratory (e.g., diabetic ketoacidosis)
    Hyperthermia or hypothermia
    Hypernatremia or hyponatremia
    Hypercalcemia
    Hypoglycemia
    Hepatic failure
    Reye's syndrome
    Uremia (also dialysis dysequilibrium, dialysis dementia)
    Pancreatitis, acute
    Myxedema

    Thyrotoxicosis
    Adrenal insufficiency
    Thiamine deficiency
Hysteria

References
1. General reference 22, p 273.
2. Plum F, Posner JB: *Diagnosis of Stupor and Coma* (3rd ed). Philadelphia: Davis, 1980.

*See also 12-G and 12-H.

12-N. Cerebrovascular Disease

Thrombosis and/or Vascular Occlusion
Thrombosis, atherosclerotic
Hypotension in presence of atherosclerotic carotid disease
    (e.g., hypovolemia, Stokes-Adams attack, myocardial infarction)
Vasculitis (especially arteritis)
    Infectious
        Subacute bacterial meningitis
        Meningovascular syphilis
        Tuberculous meningitis
        Fungal meningitis
        Protozoan and parasitic meningitis (e.g., malaria, trichinosis, schistosomiasis)
    Noninfectious
        Systemic lupus erythematosus
        Polyarteritis nodosa
        Necrotizing arteritis
        Granulomatous arteritis
        Temporal arteritis
        Takayasu's disease
Cerebral thrombophlebitis and/or venous sinus thrombosis
    (usually associated with infection of ear, sinus, face, or meninges)
Oral contraceptives
Hematologic disorders
    Sickle cell disease
    Polycythemia vera
    Thrombotic thrombocytopenic purpura
    Hyperproteinemic or hyperviscosity states
Carotid artery trauma
Radiation

Dissecting aneurysm of carotid artery (e.g., secondary to
cystic medial necrosis or dissecting aortic aneurysm)
Pressure secondary to intracerebral hematoma
Migraine syndrome
Fibromuscular dysplasia
Fabry's disease
Homocystinuria
Moyamoya disease

Embolism
Atrial arrhythmias (especially atrial fibrillation—usually with
rheumatic valvular or atherosclerotic cardiovascular
disease)
Rheumatic heart disease, especially mitral stenosis (with or
without atrial fibrillation)
Myocardial infarction with mural thrombus
Cardiac surgery, complications of (e.g., air, platelet, fat, sili-
cone embolism)
Prosthetic heart valve
Endocarditis
  Bacterial
  Nonbacterial (e.g., associated with carcinomatosis or
  systemic lupus erythematosus)
Atherosclerotic embolism from other arteries
  Aorta or carotid arteries (e.g., secondary to carotid mas-
  sage or arteriography)
  Vertebral or basilar arteries
Pulmonary vein thrombosis (especially septic or tumor em-
boli)
Fat embolism
Tumor embolism
Air embolism
Venous thromboembolism with cardiac or pulmonary right-
to-left shunt (paradoxic embolism)
Atrial myxoma
Trichinosis

Hemorrhage
Hypertension (including hypertensive encephalopathy)
Aneurysm (ruptured or unruptured)
  Saccular ("berry")
  Fusiform (atherosclerotic)
  Mycotic
Arteriovenous malformation, ruptured or unruptured
Hemorrhagic disorders (e.g., thrombocytopenia, thrombo-
cytosis, coagulopathy, disseminated intravascular co-
agulation, anticoagulant therapy)

Intracranial trauma (e.g., acute extradural or subdural hematoma, intracerebral hemorrhage)
Hemorrhage into tumor
Hemorrhagic infarction
Connective-tissue disease (especially lupus erythematosus and polyarteritis nodosa)

Reference
1. General reference 22, p 617.

12-O. Paralysis (Paresis)*

Acute (Developing in Hours)
Spinal cord injury
Spinal cord hemorrhage (secondary to vascular malformation, coagulopathy, anticoagulant therapy, trauma)
Spinal cord infarct (secondary to spinal artery thrombosis, embolism, vasculitis)
Dissecting aortic aneurysm
Aortic thrombosis
Acute necrotizing myelitis
Profound hypokalemia (serum K^+ < 2.5 mEq/L)†
Hyperkalemic or hypokalemic periodic paralysis†
Hypermagnesemia†

Subacute (Developing in Days)
Guillain-Barré syndrome
Myelitis
  Viral (especially polio, rabies, herpes zoster)
  Postinfectious (especially after measles, smallpox, chickenpox)
  Postvaccinal (especially after rabies or smallpox vaccination)
  Subacute pyogenic meningomyelitis
  Tuberculous meningomyelitis
  Acute demyelinating myelitis (e.g., multiple sclerosis)
  Acute necrotizing myelitis
Rhabdomyolysis
  Crush injury
  Excessive muscular activity
  Muscle infarction secondary to prolonged pressure and ischemia
  Polymyositis, viral or idiopathic

Diphtheritic polyneuropathy
Botulism‡
Spinal cord or epidural abscess
Spinal cord compression (e.g., secondary to tumor)

Slow (Developing over Weeks to Months)
Severe peripheral neuropathy (see 12-Q)
Multiple cerebrovascular accidents (bilateral hemiplegia)†
Polymyositis
  Infection-associated
    Viral infection
    Syphilis
    Tuberculosis
    Toxoplasmosis, other protozoan or fungal infections
    Trichinosis, other helminthic infections
  Associated with connective-tissue disease (e.g., systemic lupus erythematosus, rheumatoid arthritis, Sjögren's syndrome)
  Associated with carcinoma
  Idiopathic
Cervical spondylosis
Ankylosing spondylitis
Paget's disease
Pott's disease
Subacute combined degeneration of the spinal cord§
Neurosyphilis (syphilitic meningomyelitis, tabes dorsalis)§
Spinal arachnoiditis (e.g., following subarachnoid hemorrhage, meningitis, subarachnoid space injection)§
Chronic epidural infection or granuloma (e.g., tuberculous, parasitic, fungal)
Electrical or radiation injury of spinal cord
Multiple sclerosis
Syringomyelia‡
Amyotrophic lateral sclerosis‡

Childhood (or Young Adulthood) Onset†
Congenital
  Cerebral spastic diplegia
  Anomalies of spinal cord or vertebrae
Hereditary disease
  Werdnig-Hoffmann disease
  Muscular dystrophies
  Friedreich's ataxia
  Chronic polyneuropathies
  Niemann-Pick disease
  Tay-Sachs disease

Reference
1. General reference 22, p 718, p 1028, p 1104.

*Except as noted, all entities may produce paralysis of either legs alone or of all four extremities.
†Usually affects all four extremities.
‡Produces descending paralysis or affects arms first.
§Usually affects legs only.

12-P. Hemiplegia (Hemiparesis)

Cerebrovascular accident (see 12-N)
   Thrombosis
   Embolism
   Hemorrhage
Transient ischemic attack (TIA)
Migraine syndrome
Head trauma (e.g., brain contusion, subdural or epidural
    hematoma)
Todd's paralysis
Brain tumor (primary or metastatic)
Infection (e.g., brain abscess, encephalitis, subdural em-
    pyema, meningitis)
Nonketotic hyperosmolar coma
Vasculitis
Demyelinating disease (e.g., multiple sclerosis, acute nec-
    rotizing myelitis)
Hereditary disease (e.g., leukodystrophies)
Congenital, perinatal injury

Reference
1. General reference 22, p 37.

12-Q. Peripheral Neuropathy

Primary Motor, Acute (may have sensory involvement)
Guillain-Barré syndrome
Infectious mononucleosis
Viral hepatitis
Porphyria
Diphtheria
Toxins (e.g., organophosphorus compounds, thallium, and vaccine for rabies, typhoid, smallpox)

Sensorimotor, Subacute
Alcoholism with associated nutritional deficiency
Beriberi
Drugs, toxins
  Arsenic
  Mercury
  Thallium
  Lithium
  Gold
  Platinum
  Lead
  Industrial solvents
  Carbon monoxide
  Nitrofurantoin
  Hydralazine
  Phenytoin
  Isoniazid
  Disulfiram
  Amiodarone
Diabetes mellitus
Atherosclerosis
Vasculitis (e.g., polyarteritis nodosa, systemic lupus erythematosus, Wegener's granulomatosis, rheumatoid arthritis)
Sarcoidosis
Subacute asymmetric idiopathic polyneuritis

Sensorimotor, Chronic
Carcinoma
Amyloidosis
Paraproteinemia (especially multiple myeloma, macroglobulinemia, cryoglobulinemia)
Uremia
Beriberi
Alcoholism
Diabetes mellitus

Connective-tissue disease (especially systemic lupus ery-
thematosus)
Myxedema
Leprosy
Chronic inflammatory polyradiculoneuropathy
Hereditary disease
Charcot-Marie-Tooth disease
Dejerine-Sottas disease
Refsum's disease
Abetalipoproteinemia
Metachromatic leukodystrophy
Roussy-Lévy syndrome
Fabry's disease
Familial dysautonomia

Reference
1. General reference 22, p 1028.

12-R. Carpal Tunnel Syndrome

Fibrosis or tenosynovitis of flexor tendons
Fracture (e.g., Colles')
Occupational trauma (e.g., jackhammer or typewriter oper-
ation)
Degenerative arthritis
Wrist ganglion or benign tumor
Pregnancy
Congestive heart failure (with edema)
Amyloidosis
Rheumatoid arthritis
Scleroderma
Systemic lupus erythematosus
Diabetes mellitus
Hypothyroidism
Tuberculosis, other granulomatous diseases (e.g., leprosy,
sarcoidosis)
Gout
Paget's disease
Acromegaly
Mucopolysaccharidoses

Reference
1. General reference 22.

12-S. Typical Cerebrospinal Fluid Characteristics in Various Diseases

Condition	Pressure (cm H$_2$O)	WBCs/mm^3	Predominant type of WBCs	Glucose (mg/dl)	Protein (mg/dl)	Other
Normal	5–20	< 5	100% lymphocytes	50–75% of serum value	< 50	Lactate 10–20 mg/dl
Meningitis						
Bacterial	Usually ↑	100–100,000	85–95% neutrophils	< 40, or < 40% of blood glucose	45–500	Lactate > 35 mg/dl; positive bacterial cultures, Gram's stain, CIE, ELISA
Viral	Normal to ↑	10–500	Lymphocytes (sometimes neutrophils early)	Normal, occasionally →	50–200	Lactate < 35 mg/dl
Tuberculous	↑	50–500	Lymphocytes (occasionally neutrophils)	< 40	100–200	Lactate > 35 mg/dl; positive mycobacterial culture and/or Ziehl-Neelsen stain

	Pressure	Cell count	Cell type	Glucose	Protein	Comments
Fungal (± abscess)	Normal to ↑	25–1000	Lymphocytes	20–40	25–500	Lactate > 35 mg/dl
Neurosyphilis (meningovascular or paretic)	Normal to ↑	200–500	Lymphocytes	Normal	40–200	↑ γ-globulins, positive serologic tests (VDRL usually, FTA-ABS "always")
Herpes encephalitis	Normal to ↑	20–500	Lymphocytes	Normal, sometimes →	50–100	↑ RBCs, xanthochromia
Brain abscess*	↑ to ↑↑	20–300 (may be > 50,000 if ruptured)	10–80% neutrophils	Normal	75–100	
Neoplasm*	Usually ↑	<100	Lymphocytes	40–80	50–1000	Positive cytology

12-S. Typical Cerebrospinal Fluid Characteristics in Various Diseases (continued)

Condition	Pressure (cm H_2O)	WBCs/mm³	Predominant type of WBCs	Glucose (mg/dl)	Protein (mg/dl)	Other
Cerebral hemorrhage	Usually ↑	↑ in proportion to RBCs (may be 2000–3000)	Lymphocytes	Normal, occasionally ↓	↑↑ (< 1000)	↑↑ RBCs, xanthochromia or gross blood
Multiple sclerosis	Normal	< 100	Lymphocytes	Normal	< 100	↑ γ-globulins (> 12% of total protein); ↑ myelin basic protein

CIE = counterimmunoelectrophoresis; ELISA = enzyme-linked immunosorbent assay; ↓ = decreased; ↑ = increased; ↑↑ = greatly increased.

*If this diagnosis is suspected, lumbar puncture is contraindicated, at least until after computed tomography has been performed.

References
1. General reference 22.
2. General reference 23.

12-T. Dermatome Chart

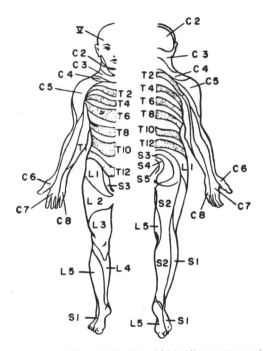

Source: Gatz AJ: *Manter's Essentials of Clinical Neuroanatomy and Neurophysiology* (4th ed). Philadelphia: Davis, 1970, p 23.

13 RESPIRATORY SYSTEM

13-A. Cough

Acute

Viral upper respiratory infection
 Pharyngitis
 Rhinitis
 Tracheobronchitis
 Bronchiolitis
 Serous otitis
Bacterial and other infections
 Tracheobronchitis
 Sinusitis, especially maxillary
 Otitis media or externa
 Pneumonia
 Lung abscess
Asthma
Inhalation of irritants
 Smoke/smog
 Noxious fumes
 Extremely hot or cold air
Pulmonary edema
Pulmonary embolism
Aspiration pneumonitis
Foreign body inhalation

Laryngeal inflammation
External or middle ear disease
Acute pleural, pericardial, mediastinal, or diaphragmatic inflammation

Chronic
"Smoker's cough"
Postviral bronchitis
Chronic bronchitis
Chronic sinusitis*
Chronic rhinitis*
  Allergic
  Perennial nonallergic
  Postinfectious
  Vasomotor
Asthma
Gastroesophageal reflux
Bronchiectasis
Neoplasms (especially endobronchial or laryngeal), malignant and benign
Lung abscess
Interstitial lung disease (see 13-N)
Recurrent aspiration
  Hiatal hernia
  Achalasia
Drug-induced
  Angiotensin-converting enzyme (ACE) inhibitors
  Beta blockers, selective and nonselective
  Amiodarone
Chronic pulmonary edema
Mitral stenosis
Chronic laryngeal inflammation or tumor
Chronic pneumonia, especially tuberculous and fungal
Cystic fibrosis
External and middle-ear disease, chronic
Miscellaneous
  Bronchogenic/mediastinal cyst
  Zenker's diverticulum
  Aortic aneurysm
  Irritation of vagal afferent nerve
  Osteophytes
  Pacemaker wires
  Chronic pleural, pericardial, mediastinal, or diaphragmatic inflammation

Psychogenic

References
1. Irwin RS, Curley FJ, French CL: Chronic Cough. *Am Rev Respir Dis* 141:640–647, 1990.
2. Braman SS, Corrao WM: Cough: Differential Diagnosis and Treatment. *Clin Chest Med* 8:177, 1987.
3. Thompson BT, Kazemi H: Pulmonary Problems. In general reference 5, p 168.

*Both diseases can cause the "postnasal drip" syndrome.

13-B. Dyspnea

Acute
Pleuropulmonary causes
   Chronic obstructive lung disease
   Asthma
   Acute tracheobronchitis
   Pneumonitis
   Pulmonary edema and congestion (see 13-L)
   Pulmonary thromboembolism
   Pneumothorax
   Pleurisy and/or pleural effusion
   Gastric or other fluid aspiration
   Noxious gas inhalation (including carbon monoxide)
   Upper airway obstruction (see 13-C)
   Collapse of lung segment(s)
   Foreign-body aspiration
   Chest trauma
      Pulmonary contusion
      Rib fractures
      Flail chest
Nonpulmonary causes
   Psychogenic disorders (e.g., anxiety)
   Decreased inspired oxygen tension (e.g., at high altitude)
   Acute neuromuscular dysfunction
   Shock
   Fever
   Acute anemia
   Increased intracranial pressure
   Metabolic acidosis
   Cardiac tamponade

Chronic
Pleuropulmonary causes
  Chronic obstructive pulmonary disease
    Chronic bronchitis
    Emphysema
    Cystic fibrosis
  Asthma
  Pulmonary edema or congestion (see 13-L)
  Diffuse interstitial lung disease
  Chronic pneumonia
  Pulmonary vascular disease
    Recurrent pulmonary emboli
    Pulmonary hypertension
    Arteriovenous malformation
  Malignancy
    Bronchogenic carcinoma
    Pulmonary metastatic disease
  Respiratory muscle disease
    Phrenic nerve dysfunction
    Neuromuscular disease
      Myasthenia gravis
      Poliomyelitis
      Guillain-Barré syndrome
      Muscular dystrophy
  Chest wall abnormalities
    Kyphoscoliosis
  Pleural disease
    Effusion
    Fibrothorax
    Primary or metastatic neoplasm
  Bronchiectasis
  Alveolar filling disease
    Pulmonary alveolar proteinosis
    Alveolar microlithiasis
    Lipoid pneumonia
  Lung resection
  Upper airway obstruction
Nonpulmonary causes
  Anemia
  Obesity
  Psychogenic disorders
  Ascites
  Metabolic acidosis
  Hyperthyroidism
  Arteriovenous shunt
  Congenital heart disease
  Abnormal hemoglobin

References
1. Ingram RH, Braunwald E: Dyspnea and Pulmonary Edema. In general reference 1, pp 220–224.
2. Thompson BR, Kazemi H: Pulmonary Problems. In general reference 5, p 170.
3. Mahler DA: Dyspnea: Diagnosis and Management. *Clin Chest Med* 8:215, 1987.

13-C. Wheezing

Asthma
Extrinsic
Intrinsic
Exercise- or cold-induced
Drug-induced
  Aspirin
  Beta blockers
  Acetylcysteine
  Indomethacin
  Tartrazine

Wheezing of Other Etiologies
Peripheral airway obstruction
  Bronchitis, chronic or acute
  Bronchiolitis
  Bronchiectasis
  Cystic fibrosis
  Pneumonia
Pulmonary embolism
Cardiac asthma
  Pulmonary edema (see 13-L)
Aspiration
  Foreign body
  Gastric contents
Irritant inhalants
  Toluene diisocyanate
  Sulfur dioxide
Anaphylaxis
Upper airway obstruction
  Extrinsic
    Thyroid enlargement, tumor, hemorrhage
    Lymphoma
    Edema of, or hemorrhage into, subcutaneous tissues
      of neck

Retropharyngeal edema, hemorrhage, abscess
Intrinsic
Epiglottitis
Foreign body
Tracheal fracture, stricture, tracheomalacia
Laryngeal tumor, trauma, edema, spasm
Vocal cord dysfunction or paralysis
Amyloidosis
Functional
Laryngeal dyskinesia
Large airway obstruction
Extrinsic
Mediastinal hemorrhage or tumor
Esophageal cancer
Vascular compression
Aortic aneurysm
Congenital anomalies
Intrinsic
Tracheal stricture, tumor, tracheomalacia
Pulmonary infiltrates with eosinophilia
Loeffler's syndrome
Tropical eosinophilia
Chronic eosinophilic pneumonia
Bronchopulmonary aspergillosis
Polyarteritis nodosa
Angioedema
Idiopathic
Hereditary angioneurotic edema
Carcinoid syndrome

References

1. MacDonnell KF: Differential Diagnosis of Asthma. In Weiss EB, Segal MS (eds): *Bronchial Asthma: Mechanisms and Treatment.* Boston: Little, Brown, 1976, p 679.
2. Thompson BT, Kazemi H: Pulmonary Problems. In general reference 5, p 173.
3. Hollingsworth HM: Wheezing and Stridor. *Clin Chest Med* 8:231–240, 1987.

13-D. Hemoptysis

Pseudohemoptysis
Blood of upper gastrointestinal origin
Upper airway lesions
  Epistaxis
  Gingival bleeding
  Oropharyngeal carcinoma
  Laryngeal carcinoma or other lesions
  Hereditary hemorrhagic telangiectasia
Serratia marcescens infection

Tracheobronchial Sources
Bronchitis, chronic or acute
Bronchiectasis
Bronchogenic carcinoma
Bronchial adenoma
Foreign body
Endobronchial metastatic neoplasm
Bronchial trauma
Cystic fibrosis
Broncholithiasis
Amyloidosis

Pulmonary Parenchymal Sources
Pneumonia
  Bacterial
  Tuberculous
Pulmonary embolism/infarction
Neoplasm
Lung abscess
Fungal infections (especially aspergilloma)
Lung contusion or laceration
Goodpasture's syndrome
Wegener's granulomatosis
Idiopathic pulmonary hemosiderosis
Inhalation injury (toxic gases)
Sequestration
Bronchogenic cyst
Parasitic infestation (e.g., hydatid disease)
Pulmonary endometriosis

Cardiac or Vascular Disorders
Pulmonary edema and congestion
Mitral stenosis
Aortic aneurysm
Primary pulmonary hypertension

Arteriovenous malformation
Eisenmenger's syndrome
Pulmonary vasculitis
Collagen vascular diseases
Behçet's syndrome
Pulmonary venoocclusive disease
Pulmonary telangiectasia

Hematologic Disorders
Coagulopathy
  Congenital
  Acquired, including anticoagulant therapy
Thrombocytopenia (see 8-J)

Undiagnosed*

References
1. Braunwald E: Cough and Hemoptysis. In general reference 1, pp 217–220.
2. Lyons HA: Differential Diagnosis of Hemoptysis and Its Treatment. *Basics RD* 5(2), 1976.
3. Israel RH, Poe RH: Hemoptysis. *Clin Chest Med* 8:197–205, 1987.

*Five to fifteen percent despite extensive evaluation.

13-E. Cyanosis*

Central Cyanosis
Arterial desaturation
  Decreased inspired oxygen tension
  Pulmonary disease
    Alveolar hypoventilation
    Ventilation-perfusion mismatch
    Impaired oxygen diffusion
  Right-to-left shunt
    Congenital heart disease
    Pulmonary arteriovenous fistulas
    Other intrapulmonary shunts
Hemoglobin abnormalities
  Methemoglobinemia
  Sulfhemoglobinemia
  Hemoglobin with low affinity for oxygen (e.g., hemoglobin
    Kansas)
Pseudocyanosis
  Polycythemia vera
  Argyria
  Hemochromatosis

Peripheral Cyanosis
Reduced cardiac output
Cold exposure (including Raynaud's phenomenon)
Arterial obstruction
Venous stasis and/or obstruction

References
1. Braunwald E: Cyanosis, Hypoxia, and Polycythemia. In general reference 1, pp 224–228.
2. Guenter CA: Respiratory Function of the Lungs and Blood. In Guenter CA, Welch MA (eds): *Pulmonary Medicine.* Philadelphia: Lippincott, 1977, p 124.

*Indicates ≥ 5 gm of unsaturated hemoglobin or ≥ 1.5 gm of methemoglobin present.

13-F. Pleuritic Pain*

Chest Wall Disease
Bony thorax
   Costochondritis (Tietze's syndrome)
   Rib fracture or tumor
   Fractured cartilage
 • Periostitis
   Periosteal hematoma
   Xiphoidalgia
• Thoracic spondylitis due to arthritis, infection, trauma
Soft tissues
   Infection
• Muscle spasm (intercostal or pectoral)
   Myositis (see 11-D)
   Fibromyositis
Neural structures
   Intercostal neuritis
   Herpes zoster
   Neurofibromatosis
   Causalgia
   Anterior chest wall syndrome

Pleuropulmonary Disease†
Infectious pleuritis, especially viral
Idiopathic pleurodynia
 › Pulmonary embolism and infarction
Pneumonia
Pneumothorax
Trauma
Neoplasm
   Primary
   Metastatic
   Direct invasion
‒ Immune-mediated disease, especially:
 • Systemic lupus erythematosus
 › Postcardiac injury syndrome
 • Rheumatoid arthritis
 › Vasculitis
Diaphragmatic irritation
   Pancreatitis
   Abscess: subphrenic, splenic, hepatic
Asbestosis
Uremic pleuritis
Radiation pleuritis
Familial polyserositis
Middle lobe syndrome

Mediastinal Disease
Pneumomediastinum
Mediastinitis
Esophageal perforation
Esophageal variceal sclerotherapy
⸗Pericarditis
Tumor, primary or metastatic

References
1. Reich NE, Fremont, RE: *Chest Pain: Systemic Differen-tiation and Treatment.* New York: Macmillan, 1961.
2. Thompson BT, Kazemi H: Pulmonary Problems. In gen-eral reference 5, pp 171–173.
3. Donat WE: Chest Pain: Cardiac and Noncardiac Causes. *Clin Chest Med* 8:241–252, 1987.

*Pleuritic pain is defined as pain accentuated by breathing, coughing, or sneezing.
†Most of the disorders that cause exudative effusions also cause pleuritic pain. See 13-G for a more complete list.

13-G. Pleural Effusion: Exudate

Exudative Pleural Effusion
Infection
  Bacterial
    Empyema
    Parapneumonic effusion
  Tuberculous
  Viral
  Fungal
  Parasitic
  Mycoplasmal
  Rickettsial
Neoplasm
  Direct pleural involvement
    Metastases
    Direct invasion from surrounding structures
    Primary pleural malignancy
  Indirect causes
    Lymphoma
    Ovarian neoplasm (Meigs' syndrome)
Thromboembolic disease
  Pulmonary embolism
  Pulmonary infarction

Immune-mediated diseases
  Rheumatoid disease
  Systemic lupus erythematosus
  Drug-induced lupus
  Wegener's granulomatosis
  Sarcoidosis
  Postcardiac injury syndrome
  Angioimmunoblastic lymphadenopathy
  Sjögren's syndrome
  Progressive systemic sclerosis
Intraabdominal disorders
  Pancreatitis
  Esophageal perforation
  Subphrenic abscess
  Intrahepatic abscess
  Splenic abscess
  Esophageal variceal sclerotherapy
  Postabdominal surgery
  Postpartum state
Drug-induced pleural disease
  Nitrofurantoin
  Methysergide
  Dantrolene
  Bromocriptine
  Procarbazine
  Practolol
  Methotrexate
  Amiodarone
Inhalation of inorganic dusts
  Asbestosis
Other causes
  Meigs' syndrome
  Yellow nail syndrome
  Uremic pleuritis
  Radiation pleuritis
  Myxedema
  Spontaneous pneumothorax
  Familial Mediterranean fever
  Trapped lung
  Postpartum pleural effusion
  Amyloidosis

Hemothorax
Traumatic
  Penetrating or nonpenetrating trauma
  Iatrogenic
Malignancy, especially metastatic

Anticoagulant therapy for pulmonary emboli
Spontaneous
  Secondary to bleeding disorder
  Rupture of intrathoracic vessel or aneurysm
  Ruptured pancreatic pseudocyst
  Thoracic endometriosis
  Idiopathic

Chylothorax

Traumatic
  Penetrating or nonpenetrating trauma
  Surgery
  Iatrogenic
Malignancy
  Lymphoma
  Metastatic malignancy
Idiopathic
Congenital
Pulmonary lymphangiomyomatosis
Pseudochylothorax

References

1. Connors AF, Altose MD: Pleural Disease. In Wolinsky E, Baum GL (eds): *Textbook of Pulmonary Diseases* (5th ed). Boston: Little, Brown, 1994, p 1839.
2. Light RW: *Pleural Diseases* (2nd ed). Philadelphia: Lea & Febiger, 1990.

13-H. Pleural Effusion: Transudate

Cardiac disease
  Congestive heart failure
  Fluid overload
  Constrictive pericarditis
  Obstruction of superior vena cava or azygos vein
Renal disease
  Nephrotic syndrome
  Acute glomerulonephritis
  Urinary tract obstruction
  Peritoneal dialysis
Liver disease
  Cirrhosis with ascites
Thromboembolic disease
  Pulmonary embolism*
Others
  Meigs' syndrome*
  Myxedema*
  Sarcoidosis
  Severe malnutrition (with hypoalbuminemia)
  Iatrogenic (e.g., venous catheter in pleural space)

References
1. Connors AF, Altose MD: Pleural Disease. In Wolinsky E, Baum GL (eds): *Textbook of Pulmonary Diseases* (5th ed). Boston: Little, Brown, 1994, p 1839.
2. Light RW: *Pleural Diseases.* (2nd ed). Philadelphia: Lea & Febiger, 1990.

*Most are exudates.

13-I. Pleural Effusion: Exudate Versus Transudate*

Characteristics of an exudative effusion:
Pleural fluid–serum protein ratio > 0.5
Pleural fluid lactic dehydrogenase (LDH) greater than
two-thirds of the upper limit of normal for serum LDH
Pleural fluid–serum LDH ratio > 0.6.

References
1. Light RW, et al: Pleural Effusions: The Diagnostic Separation of Transudates and Exudates. *Ann Intern Med* 77:507, 1972.
2. Light RW: *Pleural Diseases.* (2nd ed). Philadelphia: Lea & Febiger, 1990.

*An exudate will have one or more of these three characteristics; a transudate will not have any of these characteristics.

13-J. Empyema

Pulmonary Causes
Pneumonia
Bronchial obstruction
    Tumor
    Foreign body
Hematogenous spread of infection
Bronchopleural fistula
Ruptured abscess
Spontaneous pneumothorax
Bronchiectasis
Rheumatoid disease

Mediastinal Causes
Esophageal fistula
Abscess
    Lymph node
    Osteomyelitis
Pericarditis

Subdiaphragmatic Causes
Abscess (hepatic, pancreatic, splenic, retrogastric)
Peritonitis

Direct Inoculation
Postoperative
    Infected hemothorax

Leaky bronchial stump (postlobectomy or postpneumo-
nectomy)
Penetrating chest trauma
Foreign body in pleural space
Iatrogenic inoculation
Thoracentesis
Chest tube

Reference

1. Snider GL, Saleh SS: Empyema of the Thorax in Adults:
Review of 105 Cases. *Chest* 54:410, 1968.

13-K. Pneumothorax

✳ Primary spontaneous pneumothorax
Secondary spontaneous pneumothorax
Obstructive pulmonary disease
Chronic airway obstruction
✳ Asthma
Malignancy
Primary lung carcinoma
Pleural metastatic disease
Infectious disease
Lung abscess
Tuberculosis
Pulmonary infarction
Diffuse lung disease
Idiopathic pulmonary fibrosis
Eosinophilic granuloma
Scleroderma
Rheumatoid disease
Tuberous sclerosis
Sarcoidosis
Lymphangiomyomatosis
Idiopathic pulmonary hemosiderosis
Alveolar proteinosis
Xanthomatosis
Biliary cirrhosis
Pneumoconiosis
Silicosis
Berylliosis
Congenital disease
Cystic fibrosis
Marfan's syndrome

Catamenial pneumothorax
Neonatal pneumothorax
Traumatic pneumothorax
Penetrating thoracic trauma
Barotrauma
Sudden chest compression
Iatrogenic

Reference
1. Light RW: *Pleural Diseases* (2nd ed). Philadelphia: Lea & Febiger, 1990, p 187.

13-L. Pulmonary Edema

Elevated Microvascular Pressure
Cardiogenic (see 2-G, Left Heart Failure)
Volume overload (especially when associated with low
    plasma oncotic pressure)
Neurogenic
  Head trauma
  Intracerebral hemorrhage
  Postictal
Pulmonary venous obstruction
  Chronic mediastinitis
  Anomalous pulmonary venous return
  Congenital pulmonary venous stenosis
  Idiopathic venoocclusive disease

Normal Microvascular Pressure (Adult Respiratory Distress Syndrome)
Infection
  Sepsis
  Pneumonia
    Bacterial
    Viral
    Mycoplasmal
    Fungal
    Pneumocystis carinii
    Legionnaires' disease
  Miliary tuberculosis
  Toxic shock syndrome
  Malaria
Liquid aspiration
  Gastric contents

Water (near-drowning)
Hypertonic contrast media
Ethyl alcohol
Shock, especially septic (see 2-K)
Multiple trauma and burns
Hematologic disorders
Diffuse intravascular coagulation
Transfusion-related leukoagglutinins
Leukemia
Unfiltered blood transfusion (controversial)
Inhaled toxic gases
Oxygen (high concentration)
Smoke
Nitrogen dioxide
Sulfur dioxide
Chlorine
Phosgene
Ozone
Metallic oxides
Acid fumes
Carbon monoxide
Hydrocarbons
Cadmium
Ammonia
Embolism
Thrombus
Fat
Air
Amniotic fluid
Acute pancreatitis
Drug overdose
Narcotics
Propoxyphene
Chlordiazepoxide
Aspirin
Ethchlorvynol
Barbiturates
Colchicine
Drug-induced lung injury (see 13-N)
Paraquat
Nitrofurantoin
Amiodarone
Immunologic injury
Goodpasture's syndrome
Systemic lupus erythematosus
Associated with high negative pleural pressure
Post-thoracentesis

Postexpansion of pneumothorax
Acute bronchial asthma
Complete upper airway obstruction (e.g., hanging)
Pulmonary lymphatic obstruction
Fibrotic and inflammatory disease (e.g., silicosis)
Lymphangitic carcinomatosis
Post–lung transplant
Miscellaneous
Acute radiation pneumonitis
Pulmonary contusion
Post–cardiopulmonary bypass
Diabetic ketoacidosis
Circulating vasoactive substance (e.g., histamine)
Dextran
Lymphangiogram dye (mechanism controversial)

Unclear Mechanisms
High-altitude pulmonary edema

References
1. Ingram RH: Adult Respiratory Distress Syndrome. In general reference 1, p 1122.
2. General reference 24, p 1954.
3. Hudson LD: Causes of the Adult Respiratory Distress Syndrome: Clinical Recognition. *Clin Chest Med* 3:195, 1982.

13-M. Respiratory Failure

Central Nervous System Disorders
Drug intoxication
   Sedatives
   Tranquilizers
   Analgesics
   Anesthetics
Vascular disorders, hypoperfusion states
   Intracranial infarction or bleeding (especially brainstem)
   Shock (see 2-K)
Disorders of the central respiratory controller
   Primary alveolar hypoventilation
   Obstructive sleep apnea syndrome
Trauma
   Head injury
   Increased intracranial pressure
Infection
   Viral encephalitis
   Bulbar poliomyelitis
Miscellaneous
   Status epilepticus
   Myxedema

Neuromuscular Disorders
Peripheral nerve and anterior horn cell disorders
   Guillain-Barré syndrome
   Poliomyelitis
   Amyotrophic lateral sclerosis
Myoneural junction disorders
   Myasthenia gravis
   Tetanus
   Curare-like drugs
   Anticholinesterase drugs
Muscular disorders
   Muscle weakness due to, for example, hypophospha-
      temia, hypokalemia
   Muscle fatigue
   Polymyositis, dermatomyositis
   Muscular dystrophies
   Myotonia

Chest Wall and Pleural Disorders
Kyphoscoliosis
Chest trauma
   Flail chest

    Multiple rib fractures
    Post-thoracotomy
  Pleural disorders
    Large pleural effusions (see 13-G, 13-H)
    Tension pneumothorax
    Massive fibrosis

Pulmonary Disorders
Airflow limitation, chronic
  Pulmonary emphysema
  Chronic bronchitis
  Asthma, especially status asthmaticus
Alveolar disorders
  Pneumonia
  Aspiration pneumonitis
  Pulmonary edema (see 13-L)
    Elevated microvascular pressure
    Normal microvascular pressure (adult respiratory distress syndrome)
    Combined or unclear mechanisms
Airway obstruction, acute
  Foreign body
  Upper airway obstruction (see 13-C)
  Epiglottitis
  Respiratory burns
  Noxious gases
  Bronchospasm, acute (see 13-C)
Interstitial disorders
  Fibrosing alveolitis
  Interstitial fibrosis and other diffuse disorders (see 13-N)
  Extensive neoplasm
Vascular disorders
  Pulmonary embolus (especially thrombus, fat)
  Obliterative vasculitis
    Primary pulmonary hypertension
    Scleroderma

References
1. Smith JP: Respiratory Failure and Its Management. In Holman CW, Muschenheim C (eds): *Bronchopulmonary Diseases and Related Disorders.* New York: Harper & Row, 1972, p 694.
2. Pontoppidan H, Geffin B, Lowenstein E: Acute Respiratory Failure. *N Engl J Med* 287:690, 743, 799, 1972.

13-N. Interstitial Lung Disease

Interstitial Disease of Known Etiology
Inorganic dusts
  Silica
  Silicates, especially asbestos, talc, kaolin, diatomaceous
      earth
  Aluminum
    Powdered aluminum
    Bauxite
  Antimony
  Carbon
    Coal
    Granite
  Beryllium
  Mixed dusts
  Metal dusts, especially titanium, tungsten, cadmium
Organic dusts (hypersensitivity pneumonitis)
  Farmer's lung
  Humidifier lung
  Bagassosis
  Many others (see reference 2)
Gases, fumes, vapors, aerosols
  Gases
    Oxygen
    Sulfur dioxide
    Chlorine gas
  Fumes
    Oxides of zinc, cadmium, copper, and others (see ref-
        erence 2)
  Vapors
    Mercury
    Toluene diisocyanate
  Aerosols
    Fats
    Pyrethrum
    Bordeaux mixture
Drugs
  Chemotherapeutic agents
    Busulfan
    Bleomycin
    Cyclophosphamide
    Methotrexate
    Nitrosoureas
    Procarbazine
    Mitomycin

Antibiotics
    Nitrofurantoin
    Sulfonamides
    Penicillin
Others
    Diphenylhydantoin
    Drugs causing drug-induced lupus
    Gold salts
    Amiodarone
    Methysergide
    Carbamazepine
    Propranolol
Poisons
    Paraquat
Infections
Radiation injury
Graft-versus-host reaction
Chronic pulmonary edema
Chronic uremia
Adult respiratory distress syndrome (see 13-L)

Interstitial Disease of Unknown Etiology
Idiopathic pulmonary fibrosis
Sarcoidosis
Collagen vascular disease
    Rheumatoid arthritis
    Progressive systemic sclerosis
    Systemic lupus erythematosus
    Polymyositis-dermatomyositis
    Sjögren's syndrome
Vasculitis
    Wegener's granulomatosis
    Lymphomatoid granulomatosis
    Churg-Strauss syndrome
    Hypersensitivity vasculitis
    Overlap syndromes
Eosinophilic lung disease
    Eosinophilic granuloma
    Chronic eosinophilic pneumonia
    Hypereosinophilic syndrome
Idiopathic pulmonary hemosiderosis
Goodpasture's syndrome
Immunoblastic lymphadenopathy
Lymphocytic interstitial pneumonitis
Lymphangiomyomatosis
Amyloidosis
Alveolar proteinosis

Bronchocentric granulomatosis
Inherited disorders
  Familial interstitial fibrosis
  Tuberous sclerosis
  Neurofibromatosis
  Hermansky-Pudlak syndrome
  Niemann-Pick disease
  Gaucher's disease
Liver disease
  Chronic active hepatitis
  Primary biliary cirrhosis
Bowel disease
  Whipple's disease
  Ulcerative colitis
  Crohn's disease
  Weber-Christian disease

References
1. Crystal RG: Interstitial Lung Disorders. In general reference 1, p 1095.
2. Crystal RG, et al: Interstitial Lung Disease: Current Concepts of Pathogenesis, Staging, and Therapy. *Ann Intern Med* 70:542, 1981.

13-O. Pulmonary Hypertension

Pulmonary Arterial Hypertension (Precapillary)
Alveolar hypoxemia with vasoconstriction
  Most causes of respiratory failure (see 13-M)
  Chronic obstructive lung disease
    Chronic bronchitis/bronchiolitis
    Emphysema
    Asthma
    Cystic fibrosis
    Bronchiectasis
  Alveolar disorders
    Pneumonia
    Aspiration pneumonitis
    Pulmonary edema (see 13-L)
    Chronic alveolar filling disorders
  Upper airway obstruction (see 13-C)
  Alveolar hypoventilation
    Neuromuscular disorders (see 11-D)
    Central nervous system disorders (see 13-M)
    Obesity

Primary alveolar hypoventilation
Obstructive sleep apnea syndrome
Chest wall and pleural disorders
Chest deformity
Kyphoscoliosis
Thoracoplasty
Poliomyelitis
Muscular dystrophy
Pleural disease (especially fibrothorax)
High-altitude pulmonary hypertension
Restriction of the vascular bed
Extrinsic
Diffuse interstitial disease (see 13-N)
Sarcoidosis
Other granulomatous diseases
Interstitial fibrosis
Neoplasm
Metastatic
Alveolar cell carcinoma
Intrinsic
Pulmonary thromboembolic disease
Thrombotic
Metastatic neoplasm
Septic
Fat
Foreign material (e.g., talc)
Amniotic fluid
Parasitic
Schistosomiasis
Filariasis
Pulmonary arteritis
Raynaud's syndrome
Scleroderma
CRST syndrome
Rheumatoid disease
Systemic lupus erythematosus
Polymyositis, dermatomyositis
Takayasu's arteritis
Granulomatous arteritis
Thrombosis due to sickle cell disease
Increased flow
Patent ductus arteriosus
Atrial septal defect
Eisenmenger's physiology
Ventricular septal defect
Sinus of Valsalva aneurysm
Decreased flow
Tetralogy of Fallot

Destruction of vascular bed (e.g., emphysema)
Primary pulmonary hypertension

Pulmonary Venous Hypertension (Postcapillary)
Cardiac disease
  Left ventricular failure (see 2-G)
  Mitral valve disease
    Mitral stenosis
    Mitral insufficiency
  Left atrial obstruction
    Myxoma or other tumor
    Supravalvular stenotic ring
    Thrombus
  Cor triatriatum
Pericardial disease
  Pericardial tamponade
  Restrictive pericarditis
Pulmonary venous disease
  Mediastinal neoplasm or granuloma
  Mediastinal fibrosis
  Mediastinitis
  Anomalous pulmonary venous return
  Congenital pulmonary venous stenosis
  Idiopathic pulmonary venoocclusive disease

References
1. General reference 24, p 1833.
2. Enson Y: Pulmonary Hypertension and Its Consequences. In Baum GL, Wolinsky E (eds): *Textbook of
   Pulmonary Diseases* (4th ed). Boston: Little, Brown,
   1989, pp 1139–1162.
3. Rich S: Primary Pulmonary Hypertension. In general reference 1, pp 1087–1090.

13-P. Mediastinal Masses by Predominant Compartment

Anterior
Substernal thyroid
Thymoma
Lymphoma
Germinal cell neoplasm (e.g., dermoid)
Ascending aortic aneurysm
Parathyroid tumor
Mesenchymal neoplasm (e.g., lipoma or fibroma)
Hematoma
Bronchogenic cyst

Middle
Lymphoma
Metastatic neoplasm (pulmonary or extrapulmonary)
Sarcoid lymphadenopathy
Infectious granulomatous disease
Bronchogenic cyst
Vascular dilatation
  Superior vena cava
  Azygos vein
  Pulmonary artery
Aortic arch aneurysm
Vascular anomaly
Pleuropericardial cyst
Lymph node hyperplasia
Mononucleosis-associated adenopathy
Primary or tracheal neoplasm
Hematoma

Anterior Cardiophrenic Angle
Pleuropericardial cyst or tumor
Foramen of Morgagni hernia
Fat pad
Diaphragmatic lymph node enlargement (e.g., lymphoma)
Pulmonary parenchymal mass
Cardiac aneurysm
Pericardial fat necrosis

Posterior
Nourogenic tumor
Meningocele
Esophageal lesion
  Neoplasm
  Diverticulum

Megaesophagus of any etiology (e.g., achalasia)
Hiatal hernia
Bochdalek hernia
Thoracic spine lesion
  Neoplasm
  Infectious spondylitis
  Fracture with hematoma
Extramedullary hematopoiesis
Descending aortic aneurysm
Mediastinal abscess
Pancreatic pseudocyst
Lymph node hyperplasia
Hematoma
Cystic lesion
  Neurenteric cyst
  Gastroenteric cyst
  Thoracic duct
  Bronchogenic cyst

Diffuse Mediastinal Widening
Bronchogenic carcinoma
Mediastinal hemorrhage
Granulomatous mediastinitis
  Idiopathic
  Tuberculosis
  Histoplasmosis
Mediastinal lipomatosis
Pneumomediastinum
Acute mediastinitis

Reference
1. Wychulis AR, et al: Surgical Treatment of Mediastinal Tumors: A 40 Year Experience. *J Thorac Cardiovasc Surg* 62: 379, 1971.

13-Q. Solitary Pulmonary Nodule

Neoplasm
  Bronchogenic carcinoma
  Metastatic malignancy
  Hamartoma
  Bronchial adenoma
  Lymphoma
  Plasmacytoma
  Amyloidosis
  Other rare neoplasms
Infection
  Tuberculosis
  Histoplasmosis
  Aspergillosis (mucoid impaction)
  Cryptococcosis
  Dirofilaria immitis
Immune disorders
  Rheumatoid nodule
  Wegener's granulomatosis
Developmental disorders
  Bronchogenic cyst
  Arteriovenous fistula
  Sequestration
  Varicose pulmonary vein
  Bronchial atresia
Other
  Pulmonary infarction
  Lipoid pneumonia
  Hematoma

Reference
1. General reference 24, p 2170.

13-R. Solitary Pulmonary Nodule: Distinguishing Benign from Malignant Lesions

	Benign	Malignant
CLINICAL FINDINGS		
Age*	< 40	> 45
Symptoms	Absent	Present
History	Tuberculosis exposure	Smoker
	Histoplasmosis exposure	Extrathoracic
	Nonsmoker	malignancy
	Mineral oil use	Prior
		malignancy
X-RAY FINDINGS		
Size	< 2 cm	> 2 cm
Border*	Smooth, well-defined	Ill-defined, lobulated
Calcification*	Laminated, "popcorn," or multiple punctate	Rare, eccentric if present
Doubling time*	< 1 or > 16 months	1–16 months

*These factors are most important in distinguishing benign from malignant lesions.
Source: Modified from Fraser RG, Paré JAP (eds). *Diagnosis of Diseases of the Chest* (3rd ed). Philadelphia: Saunders, 1989, p 1390.

13-S. Elevated Hemidiaphragm

Pseudoelevation
Subpulmonic effusion
Diaphragmatic neoplasm

True Elevation
Intrathoracic conditions
   Lobar or segmental atelectasis
   Pneumonia
   Pulmonary infarction
   Rib fracture
   Pleurisy
Paralysis or paresis due to phrenic nerve dysfunction
   Bronchogenic carcinoma or mediastinal malignancy
   Surgical or nonsurgical trauma
   Neurologic disorders
      Myelitis
      Encephalitis
      Herpes zoster
      Poliomyelitis
      Myotonia
      Serum sickness following tetanus antitoxin
      Diphtheria
   Extrinsic pressure
      Substernal thyroid
      Aortic aneurysm
   Infection
      Tuberculosis
      Pneumonia
      Empyema or pleuritis
      Infection of the neck or cervical spine
   Radiation therapy
   Idiopathic
Intraabdominal pathology
   Subphrenic or hepatic abscess
   Pancreatitis
   Other intrahepatic mass lesion, especially malignancy
   Other intraabdominal mass
   Splenic infarct
Eventration
Traumatic rupture of the diaphragm

References
1. Riley EA: Idiopathic Diaphragmatic Paralysis. *Am J Med* 32:404, 1962.
2. Felson B: *Chest Radiology.* Philadelphia: Saunders, 1973, p 421.

13-T. Factors Associated with an Increased Risk of Postoperative Pulmonary Complications

General factors
    Cigarette smoking (especially > 10 pack-years)
    Chronic bronchitis
    Obesity
    Age > 70 years
    Concomitant illness
    Alcohol abuse
Surgical factors
    Thoracic surgery (especially with resection of functional lung)
    Upper abdominal surgery
Pulmonary function
    Forced vital capacity (FVC) < 70% of predicted
    Forced expiratory volume in 1 second (FEV_1) < 70% of predicted
    FEV_1/FVC < 65%
    Forced expiratory flow from 25–75% of FVC (FEF_{25-75}) < 50% of predicted
    Maximum voluntary ventilation (MVV) < 50% of predicted
    Diffusing capacity of carbon monoxide (DL_{CO}) < 50% of predicted
Arterial blood gases
    PCO_2 > 45 mm Hg
    Hypoxemia not a reliable indicator

References

1. Gass GD, Olsen GN: Preoperative Pulmonary Function Testing to Predict Post-operative Morbidity and Mortality. *Chest* 89:127, 1986.
2. Tisi G: State of the Art: Preoperative Evaluation of Pulmonary Function. *Am Rev Respir Dis* 119:295, 1979.
3. Bendixen HH: Pulmonary Problems in the Postoperative Patient. In Fishman AP (ed): *Pulmonary Diseases and Disorders.* New York: McGraw-Hill, 1980, p 1716.

GENERAL
REFERENCES

1. Wilson JD, et al (eds): *Harrison's Principles of Internal Medicine* (12th ed). New York: McGraw-Hill, 1991.
2. Woodley M, Whelan A (eds): *Manual of Medical Therapeutics* (27th ed). Boston: Little, Brown, 1992.
3. Friedman HH (ed): *Problem-Oriented Medical Diagnosis* (5th ed). Boston: Little, Brown, 1991.
4. DeGowin EL, DeGowin RL: *Bedside Diagnostic Examination* (5th ed). New York: Macmillan, 1987.
5. Samiy AH, Douglas RG, Barondess JA (eds): *Textbook of Diagnostic Medicine*. Philadelphia: Lea & Febiger, 1987.

Acid-Base and Electrolyte Disorders
6. Maxwell MH, Kleeman CR, Narins RG (eds): *Clinical Disorders of Fluid and Electrolyte Metabolism* (4th ed). New York: McGraw-Hill, 1987.

Cardiovascular System
7. Braunwald E (ed): *Heart Disease* (4rd ed). Philadelphia: Saunders, 1992.

Endocrine/Metabolic System
8. Becker KL (ed): *Principles and Practice of Endocrinology and Metabolism*. Philadelphia: Lippincott, 1990.
9. Wilson JD, Foster DW (eds): *Williams Textbook of Endocrinology* (8th ed). Philadelphia: Saunders, 1992

Eye
10. Newell FW: *Ophthalmology: Principles and Concepts* (6th ed). St. Louis: Mosby, 1986.
11. Peymann GA, Sanders DR, Goldberg MF (eds): *Principles and Practice of Ophthalmology.* Philadelphia: Saunders, 1980.

Gastrointestinal and Hepatic Systems
12. Sleisenger MH, Fordtran JS (eds): *Gastrointestinal Disease: Pathophysiology, Diagnosis, Management* (4th ed). Philadelphia: Saunders, 1989.
13. Eastwood GL (ed): *Core Textbook of Gastroenterology.* Philadelphia: Lippincott, 1984.
14. Zakim D, Boyer TD (eds): *Hepatology: A Textbook of Liver Disease.* (2nd ed). Philadelphia: Saunders, 1990.

Genitourinary System
15. Brenner BM, Rector FC (eds): *The Kidney* (4th ed). Philadelphia: Saunders, 1991.
16. Schrier RW (ed): *Renal and Electrolyte Disorders* (4th ed). Boston: Little, Brown, 1992.

Hematologic System
17. Lee GR, et al (eds): *Wintrobe's Clinical Hematology* (9th ed). Philadelphia: Lea & Febiger, 1993.
18. Williams WJ, et al (eds): *Hematology* (4th ed). New York: McGraw-Hill, 1990.

Infectious Disease
19. Hoeprich PD, Jordan MC (eds): *Infectious Diseases* (4th ed). Philadelphia: Lippincott, 1989.

Integument
20. Fitzpatrick TB, et al (eds): *Dermatology in General Medicine* (3rd ed). New York: McGraw-Hill, 1987.

Musculoskeletal System
21. Kelley WN, et al (eds): *Textbook of Rheumatology* (3rd ed). Philadelphia: Saunders, 1989.

Nervous System
22. Adams RD, Victor M: *Principles of Neurology* (4th ed). New York: McGraw-Hill, 1989.
23. Joynt RJ (ed): *Clinical Neurology.* Philadelphia: Lippincott, 1992.

Respiratory System
24. Fraser RG, et al (eds): *Diagnosis of Diseases of the Chest* (3rd ed). Philadelphia: Saunders, 1989.

INDEX